The Complete Breast Book

June Engel, Ph.D

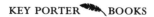

KEY PORTER BOOKS

The publisher gratefully acknowledges the assistance of the Canada Council and the Ontario Arts Council.

Canadian Cataloguing in Publication Data

Engel, June
    The complete breast book

(Your personal health series)
Includes index.
ISBN 1–55013–643–7
ISBN 1–55013–748–4 (U.S.)

1. Breast – Cancer – Popular works. 2. Breast – Diseases – Popular works. 3. Breast. I. Title. II. Series

RC280.B8E5 1996   616.99'449   C95–930374–X

The statements and opinions expressed herein are those of the author, and this book is not intended to be used as a substitute for consultation with your physician. All matters pertaining to your health should be directed to a healthcare professional.

Key Porter Books Limited
70 The Esplanade
Toronto, Ontario
Canada M5E 1R2

Diagrams: Martin Nichols
Typesetting: Heidy Lawrance Associates
Printed and bound in Canada

96 97 98 99 6 5 4 3 2 1

Contents

Acknowledgments

In preparing this book I have been immeasurably helped by many people involved in breast cancer, including survivors, activists, surgeons, epidemiologists, radiologists, dietitians, pathologists, geneticists, biologists, psychologists, psychiatrists, oncologists, nurses, social workers and family physicians across the continent.

First and foremost, I would like to thank the many people who encouraged me to write on this complex and political subject, and the many international participants I met and interviewed at innumerable conferences on breast cancer, all of whom directly or indirectly helped with the book.

I am immensely indebted to Dr. Cornelia Baines, who patiently and meticulously checked and rechecked every section of the book, and also to Dr. Pamela Chart for reviewing many sections. Those who provided me with pertinent insights include Dr. Robert Buckman, Dr. Judy Weinroth, Dr. Don Sutherland, Dr. Ida Ackerman, Dr. Rene Shumak, Dr. Charlie Katzavoulos, Natalie Parry of the Breast Cancer Exchange Project and many others.

In addition, I owe special gratitude to Dr. Roy Clark of the Princess Margaret Hospital for checking the entire manuscript *twice* and giving me many helpful revisions.

I must also particularly thank Dr. Anthony Miller, chairman of the University of Toronto's Department of Preventive

Medicine and Biostatistics, for bolstering my efforts and constructively criticizing and re-criticizing many chapters.

For advice on and checking specific sections of the book I thank Dr. Norman Boyd, Dr. David Cole, Dr. Brian Doan, Dr. Michael Drever, Dr. Eva Fishell, Dr. Vivek Goel, Dr. Wedad Hanna, Dr. Pamela Goodwin, Dr. Elizabeth Kaegi, Dr. Pamela Letts, Dr. Lavina Lickley, Dr. David Malkin, Dr. Leo Mahoney, Dr. Kathleen Pritchard, Dr. Rene Shumak, Dr. John Semple, Dr. Donna Stewart, Dr. Don Sutherland, Dr. Kathryn Taylor, Dr. Maureen Trudeau, Dr. Ellen Warner, Ms. Shirley Wheatley, Dr. Barbara Wright and Dr. Sarah Vanderburgh.

Besides advice from the medical fraternity, I could not have crafted the book without the help of many brave breast cancer survivors, activists and others who aired their views, gave me so much of their time and shed light on so many issues. Among others, they include Sharon Batt, Judy Grey, Stephanie Hall, Wendy Schain and Susan Wright.

Last, but far from least, I owe thanks to my assistant, Madeline Koch of Wordcraft Services, and to my researcher, Isolde Prince.

I dedicate this book to my friend Mary, who died of breast cancer just after giving birth to her first child, to my sister, Joyce, my daughter, Stephanie, my granddaughters, Anna and Andrea, and all the women at risk of this disease so badly in need of a cure.

Introduction

Bombarded from all sides by gloomy media messages about breast cancer, many of today's women are understandably preoccupied with the disease. However, instead of reacting with terror it's better to know the facts. Precise knowledge and understanding can be a great help in coping with and gaining control of this disease. Having breast cancer doesn't necessarily mean dying of it. Breast cancer kills fewer women than lung cancer and far fewer than heart disease. Although primarily a disease of women, breast cancer can also affect men. About 1 percent of all breast cancer occurs in men, and they too may need lumpectomies or breast removal. However, I am focusing on the disease in women.

This book grew out of a series of award-winning articles on breast cancer published in 1991 in *Health News,* a subscription health bulletin for the lay public. Another stimulus for the book was the National Forum on Breast Cancer, held in Montreal in November 1993. Jointly organized by the Medical Research Council and other medical organizations, in conjunction with breast cancer advocacy groups, this forum was a ground-breaking occasion. For the first time patients, survivors, nurses and others interested in fostering awareness participated with leading medical experts in discussing ways to combat breast cancer. It was a starting point for a new approach to the disease, with far greater consumer involvement. A flourishing survivor and activist movement has since arisen, pushing for better management of the disease and more research into ways to prevent it.

Among women in North America who live to be 85 years or older, one in ten will get breast cancer. But this much publicized figure only applies over an *entire* lifetime, not at younger ages. That's not to say that young women do not get breast cancer; some do, and some die of the disease – sometimes, tragically, mothers of young children. However, cancer is a *word*, not necessarily a death sentence. Caught and treated early, the disease can be cured. There are many women living happy lives 20, 30 and many more years after having a breast cancer removed.

Of all breast lumps investigated, only a small proportion turn out to be malignant. Having a mother or sister who has or had breast cancer does not mean that you are certain to get it; even people carrying one of the newly discovered breast cancer susceptibility genes have a 10 per cent chance of *not* getting the disease. The gene is *not* the cancer.

While understandable, random anxiety can deter women from looking after their breast health, rather than encouraging them. Fear may not only stop women from examining their breasts but may delay those who feel a lump in seeking medical attention or getting the tests that might detect an early cancer in time to prevent its spread. Helping people to dispel fear and gain control – or empowerment, to use a trendy term – is a key goal in combating breast cancer.

This book may help by explaining the difference between harmless breast lumpiness and cancer, giving a step-by-step description of what happens if cancer is suspected or found, explaining how best to get the needed information, and giving details about staging the cancer, choosing the most suitable caregivers and therapy, coping with the treatment, dealing with the medical establishment and getting breast reconstruction if desired. Throughout, the approach is practical, empathetic and "woman-centered," explaining the various choices at each stage, the treatments available, how to assess the risks and benefits of each, where and how to get advice. Besides explaining the medical management of breast cancer, the book describes ways to deal with its profound psychological and emotional impact, how to "get back a life" after the sometimes lengthy treatments, and the value of counseling, self-help or support groups and alternative or non-traditional therapies. At the end of the book there is a comprehensive list of medical and non-medical sources of advice, information and help for those who seek it.

O N E

The Healthy Breast

Many women never think of their breasts as anything other than symbols of femininity and sex appeal. Young women typically spend a lot of time wondering how to improve their breasts or make them look sexier. Most young women do not know much about normal breast structure or the signs of abnormality, or even think about the primary function of breasts – to provide milk for human infants. However, with increasing headlines about breast cancer, these shapely mounds of tissue have come under fresh scrutiny.

The recent torrent of publicity about breast cancer makes it hard to ignore the fact that breasts can harbor potentially life-threatening disease. In fact, many women have become acutely aware of – even paranoid about – breast cancer, convinced that any hint of breast lumpiness is a sure sign of it. Few know the difference between normal lumpiness and possibly cancerous lumps. To understand what is normal, one must know something about basic breast anatomy.

The Normal Female Breast
The female breast comes in a variety of shapes and sizes, but these differences have little or nothing to do with a woman's

ability to breastfeed, the amount of milk she can produce or her chances of getting breast cancer. Breasts vary so much that it's hard to say what's "normal." In most women one breast – usually the left – is slightly larger than the other. The breasts of young women tend to be firmer, denser and more cone-shaped than those of older women. Extremely large breasts can be uncomfortable and may be considered unsightly; they sometimes attract unwanted attention, or make it hard to do certain sports. On the other hand, very small or uneven breasts can stigmatize a woman and undermine her self-image. A noticeable size difference between the two breasts can make a woman painfully self-conscious. But whether large or small, conical or rounded, the main function of women's breasts is to provide milk for infants. And no matter what her breast shape or size, almost every woman who wants to can breastfeed her baby. Breastmilk is the perfect food for babies in the first few months of life.

The female breast contains functional elements – the lobes or *lobules* that produce milk, the ducts (tubes) that carry milk to the nipple – and also structural elements such as fat, connective tissue, blood vessels and lymphatic channels. (The lymph system drains off excess fluid.) The breast has about 20 lobes, each with its own tube or duct to take milk to the nipple. The nipple surface contains duct openings and each duct widens into a tiny reservoir or *lactiferous* (milk-bearing) sinus. Each duct has its own nipple opening, so that milk spurts from many openings at once. Men also have breast tissue, but no milk glands. Male breasts can also develop cancer; about 1 percent of all breast cancer occurs in men.

Except for the nipple muscles, which can make the nipple erect, the breast has no muscles of its own. It rests on the pectoral muscles of the chest wall, which lie in front of the rib cage. *Pectoralis major* is a large, triangular muscle running

Breasts Come in All Shapes and Sizes

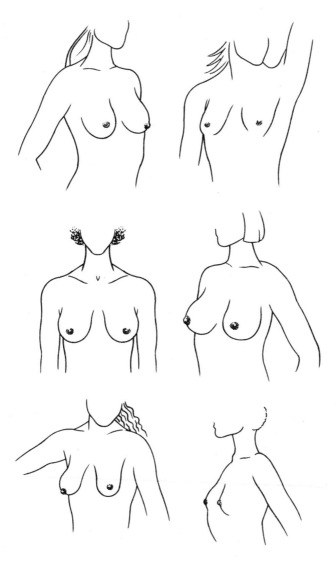

The breast is basically a modified sweat gland that starts to develop in the sixth week of fetal life, as part of a ridge called the milk line that extends from the armpit to the inner thigh on each side of the developing embryo. Ordinarily, these two ridges shrivel up before birth. As female breasts develop further, the cells change into fibrous and fatty tissue, lactiferous (milk-bearing) ducts and lobes. The network of ducts and lobes is lined by a double layer of cells.

between the collarbone, the breastbone (sternum) and the front of the sixth and seventh ribs. It helps to form the contour of the chest and to support the arm.

The skin of the nipple has a network of tiny blood vessels close to the surface, giving it a pinkish brown color. The nipple is surrounded by an area of pigmented skin, the *areola*, which varies in size, shape and color. The areola has tiny bumps on the surface; some are sweat glands, others are *Montgomery's glands*, which lubricate the nipple skin. Each breast also contains fat, fibrous tissue and *Cooper's ligaments* that help support the breast. If these ligaments get stretched by many bouts of breastfeeding or obesity, the breasts may sag or lose their shape.

Anatomy of the Female Breast Showing the Lymphatic System

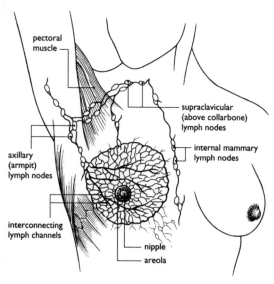

The breast is made up of irregular lobes (milk glands) with lactiferous (milk-bearing) ducts ending in the nipple. The nipple lies below the center point of the breast, and has smooth muscle, sebaceous glands that secrete lubricating material and hair follicles that give most women a little nipple hair. The lymphatics are like veins. They drain lymph (fluid) into the bloodstream, and run from the breast and nipple to lymph nodes in the armpit, base of neck and elsewhere around the breast.

Women's breasts are about one-third fat, but the percentage alters as they gain or lose weight and as they age. Very small "flat" breasts or those of very lean women may have so little fat that they feel dense (firm) and knobby, but their composition is still seldom less than one-third fat. Breast density is best assessed by a *mammogram* (breast X-ray). Recent research shows a link between breast density and breast cancer – the denser the breasts appear in mammograms, the greater the risks of breast cancer.

The lumpiness that women often feel in their breasts is a combination of milk glands, fat and fibrous tissue. As women age, milk glands are no longer needed for infant-feeding and are replaced by fat, especially after menopause. In elderly women much of the breast is fatty tissue. Hormones taken after menopause may keep the breasts more dense, delaying the normal fatty replacement.

Breast tissue receives oxygen and nutrients from blood supplied by branches of a major artery in the *axilla* (armpit) as well as the internal mammary artery, which supplies the inner half of the breast. Running alongside the arteries are corresponding veins that carry the blood back to the heart. The breast also has a *lymphatic system* – a chain of vessels rather like blood vessels that remove fluids, draining into lymph nodes (structures about the size of a kidney bean or smaller). The lymphatics play a key role in the body's defenses against infection.

Hormonal Influences on Breast Tissue

Breast tissue in women is highly sensitive to female hormones – chemical messengers that are produced by the ovaries and other tissues. Hormones circulate in the blood and affect specific "target" organs. Various hormones initiate, maintain and control the changes in female breasts during puberty,

Breast Injuries

Injuries, especially surgery or trauma (such as a hard blow), can affect breast development. If the nipple or breast tissue is injured before puberty, normal breast development can be distorted. Occasionally a skin injury – most often a severe burn – limits future breast development. Congenital (birth) conditions such as hemangiomas (a kind of birthmark) used to be treated with radiation, which damaged the nipple and young breast and often prevented further growth; this practice has been abandoned. Breast injuries do *not* increase the chances of breast cancer.

regulate the menstrual cycle, and maintain pregnancy and breastfeeding. Breast tissue is constantly changing in tune with levels of the female hormones – estrogen and progesterone. Breast cells contain certain "receptors" responsive to estrogen and progesterone, and these vary in number in different women, and at different ages. Like a "lock and key" mechanism the hormones fit onto the receptors and help regulate growth and other functions. (Pre-menopausal women have fewer hormone receptors than post-menopausal women.)

Breasts Can Give Much Sensual Pleasure

Despite the breast's primary nurturing function, most cultures eroticize breasts and consider them sexually exciting. Both the nipple and the areola have sensory nerve fibers that make them erotically sensitive; they can be stimulated to enhance sexual arousal and caressed to "turn on" women sexually. The nipple becomes erect when sexually stimulated or if an infant sucks on it. The nipple may greatly increase in size during sexual play, but typically "deflates" or becomes limp after female orgasm.

Changing Fashions

As fashions change, women's breasts are more or less openly

Structure of the Breast

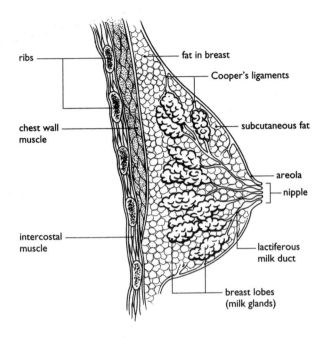

exposed, flaunted as marks of female attractiveness or hidden away as "sinful." In many cultures, breasts have a deep, almost mystical meaning. Modern Western society regards female breasts more as symbols of sex appeal than as a means of human nurturance. In striving to conform to the prevailing ideal, women push or pull their breasts into the "right shape." The heavily cleavaged look of the 1950s has given way to a lean, small-breasted image, although some fashion magazines are now portraying "ideal breasts" as somewhat fuller. Today's trends present modern women with a strange dilemma: on the one hand they are urged to display a deep, seductive cleavage, on the other they are exhorted to conform to the ultra-lean, well-exercised look.

Paradoxically, while using their breasts as sex symbols, many women are also implicitly socialized to be ashamed of them. Breastfeeding openly in public places is still curiously frowned upon among some segments of our society. As a result of such attitudes, even in our supposedly liberated feminist era, many women know little about their breasts or their primary function. Yet the thought of breasts being diseased, damaged or mutilated arouses deep instinctive fears. For these and other reasons, many women may not examine their own breasts for disease, nor do many know the normal changes that accompany the hormonal swings of the menstrual cycle, or how menopause affects breasts.

Breast Supports and Bras

In a society that eroticizes female breasts, it's no surprise that much hype surrounds breast supports and bras. The bra or brassiere is a relatively recent invention, becoming widely used only in the 1920s, as a replacement for the uncomfortable and often mutilating corsets of the nineteenth century. "However, wearing a bra is not a necessity in terms of health," notes one breast specialist. "Provided it fits, no bra is better or worse than any other. It makes no difference medically, whether a bra opens in the front or back, is padded or not, made of nylon or cotton, or has underwire supports."

Despite popular misconceptions, wearing a bra does not lead to eventual sagging. Breasts sag not because of the bra but owing to the amount of fat they contain, because of obesity or because breastfeeding has increased their size. Some women hate bras and prefer to go around braless. If a woman who regularly wears a bra decides to give it up, the breasts may hurt for a while. No need to be alarmed; it's just that the connective tissue in which the ducts and lobes are suspended is suddenly strained. Once the body gets used to being braless, the pain fades. Sports bras are increasingly popular, especially for those who jog or engage in other sports. Many women like glamorous, lacy bras that make them feel good, bolster their self-image and may add sex appeal and fun to love relationships.

Breast Changes during Pregnancy
During pregnancy, the breast grows from its usual "resting" state into a *lactating* (milk-producing) state. The lobes enlarge and develop more blood supply. Later they become laden with fat droplets and *colostrum* – the fluid that is the newborn's first food. The nipples become larger and darker in color. (Darkening of the areola is an early sign of pregnancy.)

Structural Breast Abnormalities
Sometimes the fetal milklines – present at one stage of fetal development – fail to atrophy (disappear), resulting in extra or *supernumerary* nipples anywhere along the lines. These are no cause for worry unless they are uncomfortable or embarrassing. *Amastia* – being born with breast tissue but no nipple – is a rare condition linked to developmental abnormalities of the chest. Women with this condition can have plastic surgery to create an artificial nipple that looks real but, as it lacks the nerve endings of a normal nipple, it won't respond to sexual stimulation. It has no ducts, so it cannot provide breastmilk. (See Chapter 3 for more about nipple abnormalities.)

Excessively large breasts can be displeasing and uncomfortable. They may arise because normal breast growth isn't properly "shut off." While some women welcome large breasts as sexy, others consider them a hindrance to everyday activities. Breasts that are hugely out of proportion to the rest of the body can disturb posture. They may particularly distress teenagers, who are acutely concerned about body-image and may be teased by peers. As well, women may experience extreme physical discomfort, have backache and be excluded from sports. If large breasts cause too much discomfort, women can undergo breast reduction surgery. The decision should be carefully discussed with medical caregivers, weighing the pros and cons of the operation; it may mean moving the nipple and cutting the milk ducts out, making future breast-feeding impossible.

Ultra-small breasts can also lead to self-image problems. These are often solved simply by the use of "falsies" or padded bras, but some women seek surgical breast augmentation to achieve the desired size. In the 1960s, silicone implants were welcomed by women searching for the "perfect breast." Now that the safety of silicone implants is uncertain, breast augmentation is less often done (see Chapter 17).

Poland's syndrome is a rare birth condition in which women are missing one breast; they may also have abnormalities of the arm and one side of the body. (Some women with Poland's syndrome have small but very deformed breasts.)

TWO

Benign Breast Disorders

With the increasing publicity, politics and activism surrounding breast cancer, women have become acutely aware of this disease. Understandably, many are terrified at the slightest hint of breast lumpiness. They may "think cancer" even when their breasts become *naturally* harder, lumpier or more tender because of cyclic hormonal influences. Over half the world's women occasionally have lumpy, painful and swollen breasts. One survey found that 80 percent of women in North America have some breast tenderness and benign (harmless) lumpiness, often making them miserable, anxious and fearful.

The majority of lumpy breasts never develop cancer. Most breast lumps and lumpiness are *not* cancer but just benign conditions. (The term "benign" does not necessarily mean completely harmless, but *noncancerous* – not malignant.) In pre-menopausal women under age 50 or so, less than one-tenth of breast lumps investigated (biopsied) turn out to be cancer.

Benign breast disorders such as cysts (fluid-filled sacs) and breast tenderness are most common in young women, while breast cancer is mainly a post-menopausal disease. The likelihood of a breast lump being cancer gradually increases with advancing age. "With increasing age," explains one specialist, "women move from low- to high-risk brackets for breast cancer." After menopause the chance that a breast lump is cancer rises dramatically, but even then there's a good chance that a lump will *not* be malignant. Overall, about 10 to 15 percent of breast lumps discovered and investigated turn out to be cancer.

For women who are anxious about lumpy breasts and worried that they may have cancer, the best bet is to have a thorough medical checkup and a physical breast exam by a health professional – someone they feel comfortable with, who seems competent in doing breast examinations. Specialized breast screening centers or diagnostic clinics are also good places to seek advice and referral to a breast specialist if need be.

"Women constantly seek reassurance," notes one breast surgeon. "They need reminders that breast pain and lumpiness are *not* generally a sign of cancer. It helps to lessen the anxiety if they get in touch with their breasts, examine them from time to time and demystify their fears about normal breast changes, such as the swelling or nodularity that vary with the menstrual cycle." The surgeon adds that it is not easy for caregivers to help women manage breast pain and lumpiness, because – in contrast to a solitary lump that can be removed – lumpiness is an ongoing, generalized condition that can last for years, with no easy relief or cure. "I never poohpooh or dismiss worries about breast lumpiness or cyclic mastopathy [breast pain]," she says, "but try to explain the structure of female breasts, how they fluctuate in tune with hormone levels and what such changes mean." She keeps careful tabs on women with lumpy breasts, as there is always the chance of a "dominant" or solitary lump emerging amid the general lumpiness, which needs to be investigated.

Benign Breast Disorders Include:
- *diffuse, generalized breast lumpiness and nodularity* – experienced by about 50 percent of women for a variable duration (usually a few days each month, just before the menstrual period);
- *mastalgia, or breast pain and tenderness,* either cyclical (sometimes called "cyclical mastopathy") – which occurs most often just before a period, sometimes also at the time of ovulation – or non-cyclical, which is occasionally severe and persistent enough (in 5 to 8 percent of women) to interfere with everyday life;
- *breast infections, inflammation and abscesses;*
- *breast cysts or cystic disease;*
- *papillomas* (polyps in the ducts), sometimes multiple;
- *hyperplasia,* unusually profuse overgrowth of breast tissue;
- *atypical hyperplasia* – overgrowth containing abnormal or "atypical" cells, possibly linked to increased cancer risks;
- *"dominant" (usually benign) lumps,* either solitary or multiple, such as *fibroadenomas* (benign tumors), that must be examined and distinguished from cancers;
- *nipple discharge* and other nipple problems.

General Breast Lumpiness Is Not Cancer
Much of the confusion between benign breast lumpiness and cancer has arisen through muddled concepts and fuzzy or misleading terms such as "fibrocystic disease," which is not a definite disease at all. Diffuse or general breast lumpiness ("nodularity") can occur from puberty on, but usually develops after age 30 and disappears around the time of menopause. (It may continue or reappear in those who take menopausal hormone therapy.)

Breast lumpiness is a common, noncancerous set of changes that often fluctuate in harmony with the female hormone cycle. It's most frequent in lean women, those with irregular periods and women whose mothers or sisters had lumpy breasts. It usually affects both breasts, and is most marked in the upper outer part of the breast. The lumpiness is often especially noticeable in women who also suffer severe, cyclic breast pain.

Breast Lumpiness   A Dominant Lump

diffuse thickening – no definite edge   distinct lump with definite edge

Distinguishing Breast Lumpiness from Dominant Lumps

Physicians try to distinguish general lumpiness, or "diffuse nodularity," from solitary "dominant" lumps that are distinct and palpable (felt with the fingers) – although the two can occur together. A dominant lump is a three-dimensional "mass," distinct from the surrounding tissue, but it is not always easy to tell if there is a dominant lump in generally lumpy breasts. The lump can be loose (mobile) or attached to the skin or deep tissues. It can be a fluid-filled cyst, benign tumor or cancer. Whatever it is, it needs to be medically investigated.

Managing General Breast Lumpiness
Treatment of breast lumpiness begins with reassurance that it's not likely to be cancer, and is probably due to cyclic hormone swings. Healthcare providers offer support, sympathy, education and demystification – also teaching women to do breast self-examination, looking for changes or definite lumps. They also suggest that women get regular clinical breast checkups – a physical exam by a health professional well trained in examining breasts. Once women know the lumpiness is not cancer, many will accept the condition as a fact of life and stop worrying. Those who have severe pain along with the lumpiness may wish to try medication or other treatments.

The Myth of Fibrocystic Disease
The muddled concept of fibrocystic disease has created much needless confusion and worry. Benign breast changes encompass a broad spectrum of noncancerous conditions such as lumpiness, cysts, infection, nipple discharge, blocked ducts and solitary lumps. The trouble is that these widely different conditions have been put together under misleading umbrella terms such as "fibrocystic disease."

Rumors have compounded the confusion, leading many women to believe that their so-called "fibrocystic disease" increases the risk of breast cancer. The inappropriate label of "fibrocystic disease" has caused much needless misery for women with lumpy breasts, many of whom live under a dark cloud of fear, convinced that cancer is about to strike.

Some women are persuaded to undergo useless "treatments" such as vitamin megatherapy or extreme diets, or even *mastectomy* (breast removal), to prevent the cancer they supposedly might get. The misinformation may also lead women who *do* have cancerous lumps to deny them, and pretend they're "not there."

The vague, unscientific term "fibrocystic disease" is now on the way out. In contrast to North America, European health professionals have avoided the mistake of bracketing benign breast changes under one heading. They use "fibrocystic disease" to describe only one specific symptom – breast nodularity. Other benign changes are given different names, such as mastalgia (breast pain), nipple discharge or mastitis.

In North America the term "fibrocystic disease" is now being dropped in favor of more precise terminology. Unfortunately, some of the new terms are overlapping, so a certain amount of confusion still reigns. Breast specialist and author Dr. Susan Love suggests replacing the term "fibrocystic disease" with the following categories:

- *normal physiological changes,* such as the minor tenderness, swelling and lumpiness experienced by many women during or before their periods;
- *lumpiness or nodularity* beyond the usual amount;
- *severe breast pain,* cyclical or non-cyclical;
- *breast infections and inflammations;*
- *nipple discharge* and other nipple problems;
- *dominant lumps,* such as cysts and fibroadenomas.

In 1986, the College of American Pathologists reviewed the forms of "benign breast pathology" – or departures from normal. The college concluded that only *ductal epithelial hyperplasia* (cell overgrowth) is of "clinical significance" in implying an increased risk of cancer, *and* only if the hyperplasia contains cells with "atypical" (non-typical) changes.

Breast Pain or Mastalgia

Breast pain, frequently called mastalgia or *mastodynia,* is a common complaint. (*Mast* is Latin for breast and *algia* for pain.) The tenderness can be cyclical, varying with the menstrual cycle (in about 70 percent of cases), or non-cyclical and independent of hormonal fluctuations (in 30 percent of cases). Breast pain is a frequent accompaniment to the swelling or lumpiness that occurs with the ebb and flow of female hormones, often surfacing in women during their thirties, disappearing by menopause. It can be barely noticeable, or bad enough to hinder activity and make even a hug or a tight sweater an agony. The prevalence and severity of breast pain aren't really known. Overall, 8 to 15 percent of women have pain incapacitating enough to make them seek treatment with drugs, psychotherapy or "alternative" therapies. However, studies suggest that many women with severe breast pain do not seek treatment.

Management includes a thorough medical work-up, a clear explanation of breast physiology and its dependence on hormones, and reassurance that lumpiness does not usually denote a serious disorder.

Therapies That May Relieve Severe Breast Pain:
- *a diet low in fat*, with fat intake 15 percent (or less) of total calories, and low in dairy products – recently shown to give dramatic relief to many sufferers (although it's hard to stick to such a low-fat diet);
- *oral contraceptives* (birth control pills) – either beginning to use them, or changing the contraceptives already used – helpful in young women;
- *stopping hormone replacement therapy (HRT)* in postmenopausal women; women new to HRT sometimes experience or have a recurrence of breast pain, which vanishes if they stop the hormone treatment;
- *bromocriptine* (Parlodel), which reduces the circulating levels of prolactin (a hormone that stimulates milk-

producing breast tissue). The drug helps about half of those with severe cyclical breast pain, but one-third of users develop headaches, nausea, dizziness, constipation and other side effects. Bromocriptine is rarely used for more than a few months. The drug may deform the fetus, so it must not be taken by anyone pregnant or expecting to become so. The drug is no use against non-cyclical breast pain;

- *danazol* (Cyclomen), a synthetic male hormone that lowers ovarian hormone secretion, so far the most effective medication for relieving severe breast pain. However, about a quarter of the users have troublesome masculinizing effects such as menstrual irregularity or amenorrhea (cessation of periods), weight gain, facial hair, skin oiliness, acne and a deepening voice. The side effects lessen with reduced doses; some do well by taking it on alternate days, or just in the second half of the menstrual cycle. This drug too can deform a developing fetus, so it should not be taken by those trying to get pregnant or already expecting;
- *tamoxifen*, an anti-estrogen that blocks the effect of estrogen on breast tissue, can help but its long-term safety is not established. It has some side effects such as hot flashes;
- *goserelin acetate*, given by injection, seems to help both cyclical and non-cyclical mastalgia, especially in premenopausal women. It is being studied for its possible usefulness;
- *evening primrose oil* (Efamol, Naudicelle), found in health-food stores, seems to ease breast tenderness, supposedly because it makes up for a lack of essential fatty acids (such as *gammalinolenic acid*). Studies suggest that six capsules (three grams) daily, for four months or so, reduces breast tenderness in almost half of those who try it. It can be useful for women who wish to avoid more potent medications such as danazol or bromocriptine. Evening primrose oil can

offer good relief but takes a few months to work;

- *gammalinolenic acid (GLA)*, an essential fatty acid and the key ingredient in evening primrose oil. The low toxicity of GLA, aside from mild stomach upsets, makes it a good antidote, and especially useful for those wishing to become pregnant (who should not take other drugs).

Cyclical Breast Pain

The breasts tend to be most sensitive a few days before menstruation, and less tender once the period begins. For some women, the pain starts right at ovulation, in mid-cycle, and goes on until the period begins, leaving only a couple of pain-free weeks each month. A few women have pain almost the whole month. Pain that persists longer than seven days is considered unusual and calls for medical attention. A pain chart, noting the days on which pain occurs and its severity, can help to confirm its fluctuation with the menstrual cycle, and determine the best management.

Several theories have been proposed to explain cyclical breast pain, including water retention and abnormal prostaglandin (hormone) synthesis. Psychoneurosis (mental disturbance) has also been suggested as the cause, but there is little evidence that those with breast pain are more neurotic than the general population. In 1979 a Welsh physician, Dr. Preece, studied the degree of "neurosis" in his female patients and found – to the surprise of many health professionals, who expected breast-pain sufferers to be neurotic – that breast-pain and varicose-vein patients showed similar degrees of neurosis, and definitely less than psychiatric patients.

Since it varies with the menstrual cycle, cyclical breast pain is probably linked to hormonal swings. However, there is no significant difference between female hormone levels in women with and without breast pain. In rare cases, the pain lasts beyond menopause. Post-menopausal women on hormone replacement therapy often find that the breast pain continues or resurfaces. Breast pain is quite common in pregnant women; in fact, unusual breast pain can be an early sign of pregnancy. Female hormones may induce the pain in subtle ways – perhaps as a result of stress, which is known to affect menstrual cycles. Periods can be early, late or missed when women are stressed. But the exact link between breast pain, stress and hormones awaits clarification. There is a recent suggestion that an excess of the lactation (milk-gland stimulating) hormone prolactin, secreted by the brain's pituitary gland, may be responsible. Some researchers have found that faulty regulation of pro-lactin can increase breast pain. Women who suffer breast pain also appear to be more sensitive than normal to thyroid-stimulating hormone. Low blood levels of the essential fatty acid gammalinolenic acid have been found in some women with breast pain.

The treatment of cyclical breast pain is first and foremost reassurance and support. In breast-screening clinics, about half the women seen complain of some breast pain. But once they know the pain isn't due to cancer or some other disease, simple explanations usually ease the problem. A Welsh study suggested that 85 percent of women with breast pain are more worried about the possibility of cancer than about the pain itself. Once they understand that the problem is not cancer, most are relieved and can accept or tolerate their discomfort.

Besides reassurance, the suggested treatment of cyclical breast pain includes hot baths or compresses; the use of sports bras to stop breasts from jiggling painfully; enteric-coated ASA to reduce inflammation; and above all, a diet low in fats, especially saturated fats. Breast-pain sufferers have often tried everything from ginseng tea and vitamins A, E and B complex to herbal tonics and iodine. Many remedies, such as thyroid hormones, elimination of dietary *methylxanthines* (in coffee, tea and chocolate), and vitamins E or B$_6$, have been proposed but few have any scientifically proven value. However, some treatments reportedly work in some women, despite the lack of scientific backup. Diuretics (water pills) are no longer considered useful, and may be harmful because of their general effects on the body; their use is discouraged.

Medications for cyclic breast pain include some of those already listed – danazol, bromocriptine, tamoxifen and evening primrose oil. Scientists theorize that the usefulness of unsaturated fatty acids in easing breast pain is related to their ability to replenish a dietary lack of fatty acids. Substitution of saturated dietary fat with olive oil is said to be helpful.

What to Do about Cyclical Breast Pain

- Make a pain chart to track the amount of pain and when it occurs.
- Get a thorough checkup from a health professional.
- Try painkillers such as ASA, acetaminophen and ibuprofen.
- Wear a firm bra to prevent bouncing breasts from increasing the discomfort.
- Adopt a really low-fat diet (with fats making up only 15 percent or less of total energy or calories); also limit dairy products and other sources of saturated (animal) fat.
- Decide whether you can live with the pain, or whether it is worth trying hormonal or drug treatment. Discuss this with your healthcare provider.
- If the pain interferes with daily life, ask about medications such as danazol or evening primrose oil.
- Try the contraceptive pill.
- Women with really severe pain seeking rapid relief may try bromocriptine, despite the side effects.
- Anyone on medication needs careful medical supervision.

Non-cyclical Breast Pain

Non-cyclical pain, far less common than cyclical pain, tends to occur in women in their forties and fifties. It often affects just one breast, and is less likely to be accompanied by breast lumpiness. Non-cyclical breast pain doesn't vary with the menstrual cycle but just lingers on. It is also known as "target-zone breast pain" because it's often in one specific area of the breast. Rarely, localized pain can be a sign of cancer, so it's a good idea to check it out with a physician. One cause of non-cyclical breast pain is trauma – a blow to the breast, or an operation or biopsy.

Treatment for non-cyclical breast pain is more difficult than for the cyclical variety. A thorough breast exam is the first step, and possibly also a mammogram. If there's any obvious abnormality, it can then be taken care of. Hormonal treatments are less likely to work with non-cyclical pain. Some women, however, obtain relief with the drug treatments discussed above for cyclical mastalgia. Surgically removing part of the breast doesn't work. The painful changes can recur elsewhere in the breast.

Breast Cysts

So-called "gross cystic disease" is the most frequent benign disorder of the female breast. At some time in their lives, about 7 percent of women in the Western world visit a physician or clinic because of a distinct breast lump that turns out to be a cyst. Cysts are often "palpable," or felt, as movable, perhaps roundish lumps of varying sizes. Some grow to a very large size, but most are discovered and aspirated (drained) well before that. Cysts are most common between ages 40 and 50, rare in women under 30. Some women have several at one time.

Breast cysts are basically glands or ducts that have filled with

The Caffeine Myth

In 1979, a group of researchers began to link caffeine with breast changes. Women (and medical caregivers) came to believe that avoiding caffeine might relieve lumpiness and breast discomfort, even suggesting that avoiding coffee might prevent breast cancer. Today, medical experts generally agree that there's *no* definite link between coffee and breast cancer or other breast problems; but if reducing caffeine intake seems to lessen the discomfort, why not do so?

fluid, and stretched, forming a lump that can be painful. Ultrasound examination can help determine whether a lump is fluid-filled (a cyst) or solid.

The usual treatment for a breast cyst is to drain the fluid by fine-needle aspiration (FNA), a simple procedure done in the doctor's office. Once drained, most cysts don't refill with fluid, but a significant number come back. The fluid removed from cysts varies from pale yellow to muddy brown or green. If the fluid withdrawn is bloody, it is sent for cytological (cell) examination. A surgical biopsy is usually done if the aspirated fluid is bloody or if a cyst or cysts persistently recur, after several drainings. Some cysts return many times in one spot.

Very occasionally, after a cyst is drained, a cancerous lump obscured by the cyst is uncovered in the same location. This is rare, and usually occurs in post-menopausal women.

Dominant Breast Lumps

A distinct or "dominant" lump feels different from the general nodularity or lumpiness of the surrounding breast tissue. It may or may not be cancerous. Dominant lumps are rarely malignant in women under age 30, but are increasingly likely to be cancerous with advancing years.

All dominant or solitary breast lumps *must be medically investigated*, even though most are benign. Besides physical examination, the work-up may include ultrasound (in young women), mammography and needle aspiration or surgical biopsy. Mammograms are not 100 percent foolproof, but together with a clinical exam and needle aspiration they can help to determine whether a breast lump is cancerous.

Benign Fibroadenomas

Found mostly in women under age 40, fibroadenomas are dominant but benign lumps that are usually painless. They are normal variants of breast growth and account for about 12 percent of all lumps found in women's breasts. They can be distinctly felt as firm, smooth, usually movable lumps. They do not indicate any extra risk of cancer, and do not usually recur. Hormonally dependent, these lumps swell and diminish in tune with menstrual cycles.

It is not unusual to find several fibroadenomas in one woman. They often regress and fade away, but they can calcify and show up on a mammogram. Assessment with clinical examination, fine-needle aspiration or core biopsy and mammography – perhaps also ultrasound – can often determine whether the lump is benign or cancerous. Mammograms would certainly be advised for any breast lumps found in women at high risk of breast cancer (such as those with a strong family history of early disease).

Formerly, all breast fibroadenomas were removed for fear of missing a cancer. But there is now disagreement about whether or not they all need to come out, especially if a needle biopsy shows no sign of malignancy. If found to be non-cancerous, the fibroadenoma may simply be left in place and followed every few months. Any that increase in size need removal, and in women over age 40 they should be removed because of the increasing risk of cancer. However, given a choice of "observation or excision," many women of all ages prefer to have the lump out. In one study, 5 percent of fibroadenomas assumed to be benign turned out, in fact, to be cancerous.

Phylloides Tumor (Cystosarcoma Phylloides)

A very rare condition, found mainly in women aged 40 to 50, this is a rapidly expanding tumor that becomes malignant in 15 to 25 percent of cases. Since they vary from benign to malignant, these tumors need wide excision and complete removal to make sure they will not recur.

Intraductal Papilloma and Papillomatosis

Usually harmless, and typically found in women aged 40 to 60, papillomas are tiny, benign polyps or wartlike growths in the breast ducts that may produce a watery (sometimes bloody) nipple discharge. For example, one 40-year-old woman who found a bloodstain on her nightie assumed it came from an accidental scratch, but when it reappeared night after night, even on clean nightwear, she became alarmed and consulted her doctor. More blood emerged on squeezing the nipple, and the problem was diagnosed as ductal papilloma. The affected ducts were surgically removed on an outpatient basis to test for malignancy. Fortunately, no signs of cancer were found. Even if many in number, papillomas are usually innocuous, but multiple papillomas, although uncommon, are thought to slightly increase breast cancer risks.

Papillomas (Growths) Inside a Duct

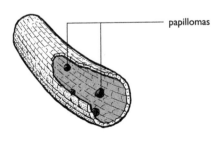

papillomas

Breast Infections, Abscesses and Inflammation

Breast infections fall under four main categories: lactational mastitis, breast abscesses, non-lactational mastitis and subareolar abscesses.

Lactational Mastitis

Lactational mastitis (inflammation) occurs in breastfeeding women. Ducts blocked with milk that doesn't flow well may trap and encourage bacterial growth. An infection can set in, causing a red, hot, swollen and painful breast. The remedy is to try to unblock the duct and get rid of the infection with massage and warm soaks. If the infection persists, antibiotics are used. Nursing at the affected breast can continue, and is encouraged; it stimulates milk flow and helps oust the infection.

Breast Abscess

A breast abscess develops from a breast infection. An abscess is a collection of pus – somewhat like a boil – that needs to be drained. If it's extremely small, the pus can be aspirated with a needle. If it's bigger, the physician will make an incision large enough to let the pus drain out, usually with local anesthetic. Some surgeons suggest that women with breast abscesses stop breastfeeding, but there's no scientific reason to give up breast-feeding. (For more information, consult La Leche League or your local breastfeeding clinic.) Although unusual, a breast abscess can arise in a non-lactating woman. And an abscess *can* mask cancer – a rare possibility that must be considered.

Non-lactational Mastitis

Non-lactational mastitis or breast infections are most likely to appear in women who have had lumpectomies followed by radiation, or those who have diabetes or defective immune systems. As one expert explains, "this type of infection usually

Subareolar Abscess

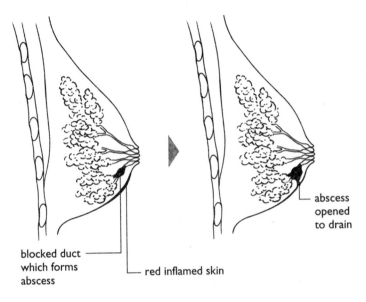

blocked duct which forms abscess

red inflamed skin

abscess opened to drain

affects the breast skin – which becomes red, hot and swollen, accompanied by high fever. It is treated with antibiotics, usually penicillin, possibly with brief hospitalization."

Skin boils (usually staphylococcal infections) can form on the breast skin, as on other parts of the body, and are treatable with antibiotics.

Subareolar or Nipple Abscesses

A subareolar abscess occurs under the areola. It is a red, hot, sore area at the nipple edge that can look and feel frightening.

This type of abscess requires immediate attention. Caught early, it can be cleared up by antibiotics alone, but otherwise it may need drainage via an incision, under local or general anesthesia. These abscesses can be very bothersome and tend to recur.

Other Breast Inflammation

A *galactocele* is a dilation and inflammation of a duct in the lactating breast. With this condition, even gentle breastfeeding causes pain and soreness, perhaps allowing bacteria to penetrate the skin. Breast infection may result.

Chronic periductal mastitis – associated with blocked ducts full of stale secretions – is an inflammatory breast disorder that usually occurs after age 45.

Mammary duct ectasia is a benign condition, not common after age 40. The breast ducts become distended and clogged with cellular debris and sticky secretions, leading to inflammation and perhaps also inverted nipples. Ectasia can be very painful and can cause subareolar abscesses, skin retraction and ulceration, with intense inflammation, redness and swelling. Treatment is usually local surgical excision to remove the affected area. The condition can recur, and some women resort to mastectomy as a final solution.

Mondor's disease, or "phlebitis of the breast," is due to an inflamed vein perhaps caused by a blow or other trauma. It produces a surface lump or groove running along the breast, with pain and a "pulling" sensation, and can also cause chest pain. The condition is self-limiting, but heat can relieve it.

Fat necrosis is an inflamed lump in the breast's fatty tissue, commonly arising from a blow or trauma to the breast. It requires a biopsy to rule out cancer. It usually occurs in the top breast layers, often near the nipple, and is more frequent in those with large breasts and in women over age 50. The fatty lump may get bigger, remain unchanged or develop into a large lump that is hot, reddened and inflamed, with some skin-dimpling. Some disappear. For bothersome fat lumps, local excision is the answer, with tests to make sure the lump is not cancerous. (Lumps assumed to be fat necrosis can hide a cancer beneath.)

Which Benign Breast Disorders Increase Cancer Risks?

The evidence for links between benign breast changes and cancer remains hazy. Of the broad spectrum of benign breast conditions, only a few – high breast density, atypical epithelial hyperplasia (tissue overgrowth containing "atypical" cells), gross (huge) cysts and ductal papillomatosis (multiple duct growths) – are currently believed to increase the risk of breast cancer.

Although women with dense breasts won't necessarily develop breast cancer, analysis of the Canadian National Breast Screening Study (NBSS) results suggests that they have five to six times the average risk. This knowledge may help in early cancer detection, but the breast density can't be determined simply by feel – it only shows up on the mammogram. Lean pre-menopausal women tend to have dense breasts; having children at an early age tends to reduce breast density. (See also Chapter 11.)

Accumulating evidence suggests that some breast cancers may be the end result of a *continuum of change* from benign hyperplasia to atypical hyperplasia to carcinoma. But while it seems that some cancers arise from benign atypical hyperplasia, the progression is not inevitable. Only a small number of those with atypical breast changes go on to develop cancer. If atypical hyperplasia occurs together with known early breast cancer risk factors (such as breast cancer in close relatives, or very dense breast tissue), the risk can be higher. Women with atypical hyperplasia need careful follow-up.

As to whether very large breast cysts elevate breast cancer risks – the matter remains unsettled. Studies suggest there may be a slightly greater risk in women with large cysts easily felt by hand, but the extent of the risk remains unclear.

How Hyperplasia Can Progress to Cancer

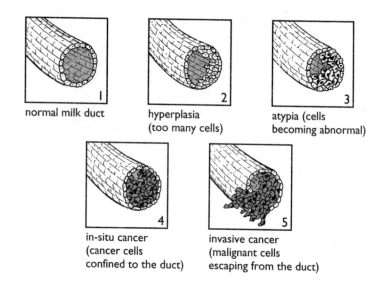

normal milk duct

hyperplasia
(too many cells)

atypia (cells
becoming abnormal)

in-situ cancer
(cancer cells
confined to the duct)

invasive cancer
(malignant cells
escaping from the duct)

Fibroadenoma has long been assumed *not* to raise breast cancer risks, but very recent studies indicate that certain types of fibroadenoma may be associated with a modestly increased risk, particularly if they contain atypical cells.

Women known to be at very high risk of breast cancer – for example, women with dense breasts, those who have atypical hyperplasia and those with several close relatives (mothers, sisters, grandmothers) who have had pre-menopausal breast cancer – may wish to take preventive steps, and can offer to participate in clinical trials such as the International Prophylactic Tamoxifen Trial. (See Chapter 20.)

THREE

Nipple Problems

There are a number of disorders and abnormalities that can affect the nipple itself. Most are not serious.

Nipple Discharges

Nipple discharges are quite common and can be an obvious drip, a rope of fluid or crusts forming on the nipples. With the rising popularity of breast self-examination, more women and their physicians are discovering that squeezing the nipple produces a few drops of fluid. At one U.S. breast clinic, nipple secretions were noted in 83 percent of breasts that were squeezed or suctioned. Most women of reproductive age will exude a little liquid if the nipple is squeezed really hard. Discharge from both breasts is less worrisome than one that emanates from a single nipple.

Nipple discharges can arise from sexual stimulation, hormonal swings or use of certain medications. Women taking birth control pills, blood pressure drugs such as methyldopa or major tranquilizers such as chlopromazine tend to notice more discharge because these medications increase the levels of the hormone prolactin. Nipple discharge may be a sign of duct ectasia (see Chapter 2) or, occasionally, of breast cancer. In contrast to discharges that occur on squeezing the nipple, one that is spontaneous, persistent and non-lactational, coming directly out of mammary ducts on the nipple surface, may mean underlying disease and needs medical attention, especially if it is bloody. In pre-menopausal women, a spontaneous nipple discharge rarely heralds any serious disorder, especially if it squirts from several ducts. "Nipple discharge does not usually signify trouble," says one breast specialist, "unless it is bloody, copious and milky, or comes from a single opening. Women with pussy, bloody, multicolored, sticky or purulent nipple discharges should seek medical attention and get a thorough breast exam."

Several conditions can produce false or pseudodischarges on or near the nipple surface. These conditions include inverted nipples, eczema, traumatic (frictional) erosion (including jogger's nipples), and herpes simplex infections. Only about 4 percent of all spontaneous, one-sided, bloody discharges are due to cancer. Pussy, milky, multicolored or sticky discharges are not generally related to cancer. But a profuse milky discharge in a non-lactating woman may indicate a pituitary tumor and calls for a thorough hormone assessment.

A pussy discharge due to a breast infection is one-sided and spontaneous, accompanied by pain and inflammation. It most commonly occurs in women with post-birth mastitis, lactational mastitis or breast abscesses. If there is an abscess, incision and drainage must be done, and a biopsy of the abscess wall should be performed to rule out underlying cancer. Treatment is with appropriate antibiotics (based on the results of a lab culture).

In a post-menopausal woman, a pussy or bloody discharge may indicate the presence of an *intraductal papilloma* (a wartlike growth) in a breast duct that becomes raw and bleeds, duct ectasia (narrowed ducts) or sometimes cysts.

Galactorrhea, a condition seen in women who are not breastfeeding, can cause a spontaneous, multiple-duct, milky discharge in the childbearing years. Most common after pregnancy, it can last a year or two, or longer. Galactorrhea may be triggered by excess production of prolactin, either directly, from the pituitary gland, or indirectly, through endocrine (hormone) abnormalities or from certain drugs (such as oral contraceptives, marijuana and tranquilizers). Pituitary tumors may be the cause, and can occur at any age, increasing prolactin levels. The condition can be less worrying than it sounds: often it's a tiny tumor that may not require surgery. A neurosurgeon and an endocrinologist together need to check this out. Use of bromocriptine can block excess prolactin production. Serious galactorrhea is often associated with *amenorrhea* – cessation of periods. Treatment is with tricyclic antidepressants, methyldopa or oral contraceptives.

Treating Nipple Discharge

In evaluating the nature and cause of a nipple discharge, the physician will determine whether it is due to hormonal variation or some pathological (abnormal) condition. Placing a drop of the discharge on a card and adding a chemical called guaiac can give a clue. If the sample turns blue, it contains

---

When to Worry about Nipple Discharge:
- when it's persistent and only on one side;
- when it's spontaneous, oozing out by itself without squeezing;
- when it happens often;
- when it's sticky, like eggwhite, or bloody;
- when it occurs after menopause and is pus-filled or bloody.

blood (which may not be visible to the naked eye). As with a Pap smear, which tests the vaginal discharge, a smear of the nipple discharge is put on a glass slide and sent to the lab for cytology, to have the cells examined. Although far from 100 percent accurate, the test may indicate whether the discharge contains any abnormal or cancerous cells.

Women over age 30 may be sent for a mammogram to see if there's a tumor underneath the duct producing the discharge. A ductogram may also be done: the radiologist threads a fine plastic catheter into the duct, squirts dye into it and takes a picture. The procedure sounds uncomfortable, but it's not – the duct is already open and the discharge has widened it. The ductogram provides a visual "map" for tracing the source of the discharge.

A specialized type of breast biopsy may follow, done under local anesthetic, on an outpatient basis. A tiny incision is made at the edge of the areola, which is then flipped up, and the abnormal duct is located and removed. Sometimes X-ray localization helps to pinpoint the affected duct; a fine wire is passed into the duct to locate the precise area to be removed.

In women past childbearing age, or those who are sure they do not want to breastfeed, the surgeon may remove all the ducts instead of just one, to make sure the problem duct isn't missed. Even if they're not all removed, the ducts are so close to each other that the removal of one can cause scarring that will interfere with future breastfeeding on that breast.

Other Nipple Problems

Nipple dryness or itching does not usually indicate a severe problem, especially if both nipples itch. It may just be due to dry skin or an allergic reaction to the bra or other underwear, or the detergents they are washed in. Pubescent girls with growing breasts often experience itching as the skin stretches.

Other than skin dryness, scientists don't know what causes itchy nipples. If they are bothersome, calamine lotion or other anti-itch medications may help.

A *scaling nipple* may indicate Paget's disease, a condition associated with an underlying cancer, which produces ulcerated, scaling and itchy skin, often confused with eczema. If there is heavy scaling on one nipple, and the ulceration looks like an open sore and doesn't go away with standard eczema treatments, it should be medically checked out. Note that in eczema the scaling is usually on both sides, and is in the areola *around* the nipple (sparing the nipple), while in Paget's disease the nipple itself scales and ulcerates. To examine the nipple skin for Paget's disease, a sliver is shaved off and sent for examination, or a "punch" biopsy can be performed on a small section of the nipple skin. Paget's disease can be associated with cancer elsewhere in the breast, and may extend down from the nipple into the breast tissue itself – a more aggressive form than that which affects the nipple only. The treatment is surgery to remove the cancer, nipple and areola, followed by a course of radiation. Mastectomy may be needed if the tumor penetrates deep into the breast.

Nipple Abnormalities

Polythelia – Multiple or Supernumerary Nipples

"Polythelia" is from the Greek meaning "many nipples." This is a common anomaly, present at birth in 1 to 5 percent of the population, and more frequently found on the left side of the body than on the right. In males it is sometimes associated with gynecomastia (excessive breast growth).

The supernumerary or multiple nipples may occur with or without glandular breast tissue, with or without areolas; indeed there may be several complete breasts, generally situated between the chest and the umbilicus along the "milk line" that runs down to the groin on each side of the body. Supernumerary nipples usually occur below normal breasts, although they have been reported in the vulva, neck, back and thigh. Occasionally there is an extra breast, or areola, with no nipple.

One author in ancient Rome described a "beautiful woman, with four breasts in a row, all producing abundant milk." Anne Boleyn, one of Henry VIII's wives, reputedly had multiple nipples. Astarte, the Phoenician goddess of love, was also said to have many breasts and nipples. Darwin considered extra nipples to be throwbacks to the multi-breasted mammals from which humans descended. The nipples are often quite small, and may go unnoticed or be mistaken for moles. Extra nipples usually swell in tune with the menstrual cycle and secrete milk in women who are breastfeeding, but generally cause no special inconvenience, unless the woman considers them esthetically displeasing.

Athelia – Missing Nipples
Athelia is rare, and usually but not always associated with amastia, absence of breasts – an exceedingly rare congenital malformation. In cases where there's no breast tissue, the pectoral muscle may also be deficient. Athelia can be corrected through techniques similar to those employed in post-mastectomy nipple reconstruction, with plastic surgery, using a composite graft from the other nipple, or multiple local flaps (grafts) plus tattooing dyes to correct the color.

Inverted Nipples
Inverted nipples occur in at least 2 percent of women. Many women seek surgical correction, not only for esthetic reasons but also to improve the chances of breastfeeding their babies. Inverted nipples may be congenital (present at birth), or may

appear following a breast infection (mastitis) or breast reduction surgery or because of scarring after breast biopsies. Often they are inverted because of scar tissue that holds them down.

Surgery to correct the nipple inversion may simply mean releasing the scar tissue. But the operations do not always succeed, as the inversion may come back. Before embarking on corrective surgery, it is essential to differentiate an "umbilicated" nipple (which can be momentarily extracted from its inverted position) from an "invaginated" nipple (which cannot be forcefully made to stand up). Breastfeeding is usually possible in women with umbilicated nipples, given enough perseverance and some help from nipple shields; a suction pump may also be required. The woman with invaginated nipples will find it difficult or impossible to breastfeed.

To correct an inverted nipple, surgery releases all the fibrous and ductal systems that hold it down; but for women with inverted nipples who want to breastfeed, surgeons must take care not to damage the milk ducts.

Correcting an Inverted Nipple

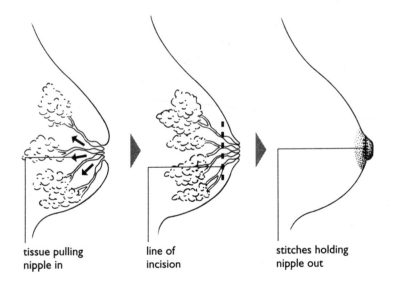

tissue pulling
nipple in

line of
incision

stitches holding
nipple out

Bifid, Fissured and Imperforate Nipples

Bifid, fissured and imperforate nipples are very rare and produce no adverse functional effects. In the bifid, or duplicated, nipple, two nipples share one areola. Fissured nipples are a milder form of polythelia; the nipple is usually small and weak, and can irritate a breastfeeding baby's palate and cause vomiting. Flattening the nipple by cutting the skin from the borders above and below can remedy the condition. In one reported case, the lactiferous duct opened between the nipples and the woman couldn't breastfeed.

FOUR

Detecting Breast Cancer Early

A lthough understandably terrifying, finding a breast lump doesn't mean you have cancer – and having breast cancer doesn't necessarily mean having a mastectomy, and it isn't a death warrant. There are thousands of women leading healthy lives 10, 20, 30 or many more years after removal of a malignant breast tumor. Breast cancers that are small when found are more likely to be curable, provided the cancer is treated before it metastasizes (spreads).

Early Detection Is Vital

To detect breast cancer early, women aged 25 and over should have regular breast examinations by a skilled health professional and should examine their breasts once a month for unusual changes. Women over age 50 should have a mammogram (breast X-ray) at an *accredited facility* at least every two years.

In contrast to benign breast lumps, cancerous tumors may invade and destroy surrounding tissues. Cancer cells can escape the tumor and travel to distant sites, when they form *metas-*

tases (secondary or spreading cancers). Some breast cancers grow fast and rapidly penetrate nearby tissues – sometimes within months, especially in young women – while others take 10, 20 or more years to become invasive. Some never spread.

Ways to Detect Breast Cancer
Breast cancer can be detected by:

- breast self-examination (BSE);
- regular physical examination by a health professional;
- mammography.

The combination of skilled physical examination, women's own "breast vigilance" or breast self-examination plus mammography detects most breast cancers. Breast cancer is most often discovered by women themselves when they notice a lump or thickening.

Breast cancer incidence (the number of new cases found per year) increases *progressively* with advancing age. In women under age 40 or so, 70 percent of lumps biopsied are benign, but by age 70 almost three-quarters of the lumps biopsied are cancerous. Women who have cancer in one breast are at increased risk for malignancy in the other.

To detect the cancer early and reduce risks, women are advised to examine their breasts monthly and to have regular medical breast checkups. Those over age 50 should have mammograms every two years.

The lumpiness and breast swelling that many women experience, especially just before a period, are *not* cancer. The tiny swellings or normal bumps around the nipple, called Montgomery's glands (see Chapter 1), are also not cancer. However, any *new or unusual* breast lump, thickening or obvious change seen in one or even both breasts should be medically checked.

Warning Signs of Breast Cancer:
- a new lump or thickening of tissue felt in the breast;
- changed size, shape or contour of one breast or nipple;
- inversion (drawing in) of the nipple;
- nipple scaling (flaking);
- skin *erythema* (redness), thickening or ulceration;
- lump or swelling in the armpit;
- persistent localized breast pain (an unusual sign of breast cancer);
- dimpling/puckering of the breast skin;
- spontaneous bloody discharge from the nipple (rare).

Swelling in the armpit can also be an occasional sign of cancer and should be reported to the doctor.

Breast Examination by a Health Professional

Although it misses some cancers, regular physical breast examination performed in a thorough, consistent manner by a qualified health professional is crucial for early cancer detection. The breasts should be examined as part of a routine medical checkup by the woman's family physician, gynecologist or other healthcare professional, especially over age 50. But some women are reluctant to have their breasts examined, perhaps for fear of finding cancer. And not all physicians are comfortable about palpating women's breasts for abnormalities. In today's confrontational climate, some physicians may fear that a breast exam will invade a woman's privacy or trigger charges of sexual abuse. Some are not well trained or adept in examining a woman's breasts. They may have had little medical-school training in this area, and may not probe the breasts thoroughly.

Nevertheless, breast palpation (examination by hand) is not foolproof; some very large, diffuse cancers are completely missed by manual examination, even by the most experienced of breast examiners. One U.S. research team found that physical examination correctly identified only 58 percent of palpable cysts. Other researchers document a surprising lack of agreement between experienced breast examiners about physical findings.

Age also plays a role. The chance of a lump being cancer in women under age 25 is very small, but it is also more difficult to detect cancer in the dense breasts of young women. Near or past menopause, breasts become fattier and less dense, making it easier to feel cancerous lumps and image them on mammograms.

Women who think their breasts are not being regularly and adequately examined can seek advice from another physician,

Clinical Breast Examination

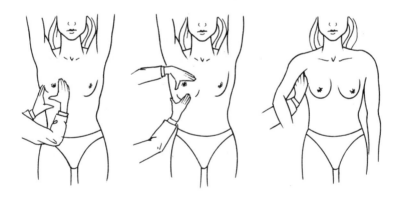

In a clinical breast examination, a health professional palpates the breasts in a consistent, systematic pattern.

or from a local breast-screening or diagnostic center or hospital breast clinic, or ask for referral to a specialist.

Mammograms

If the physical breast exam reveals a suspicious change, the next step will probably be a mammogram (breast X-ray) to decide on the need for biopsy. Mammography remains today's most sensitive method for detecting early breast cancer. Together with physical examination, it is the standard way to screen for breast cancer.

Yet, despite their increased risk, less than half the women in North America over age 50 are getting the recommended mammograms. They may avoid mammograms because they fear that the process will hurt, or that the X-rays will "travel round the body and cause damage." (See chapters 5 and 6 for more on mammography.)

Why Should I Do Breast Self-Examination?

Many breast cancers (about 75 percent) are still found by women themselves. Women know their breasts better than anyone else, so they are most likely to notice a change. Some women always feel some nodularity or lumpiness – that's their "normal" breast texture – but they may still notice a new or changed look or "feel." Occasionally breast cancer is discovered because it hurts, but that is the exception rather than the rule. More often, a cancerous lump gives no clue of its presence until the woman or the doctor examining her notices it, or it shows up on a screening mammogram.

The key to the success of breast self-examination is to report any change immediately. Naturally, finding a new lump can send shivers of fear through a woman. She may probe and feel the suspicious spot over and over again to test whether it's her imagination or whether it's really there. Studies show that women often delay reporting a lump to their physician, sometimes for weeks, not so much through neglect or ignorance but because of apprehension that it may be cancer.

It may help women not to panic on finding a lump if they remember that most of the breast abnormalities investigated turn out *not* to be cancer. "As some measure of reassurance," says one breast surgeon, "and to encourage women to see their doctors early about a breast problem, I remind them that of all breast lumps we investigate or biopsy, the majority are benign, non-cancerous changes."

Breast self-examination, or BSE, can be a valuable adjunct to clinical breast exams and mammography in spotting breast cancer early, but only if women swiftly report the changes they find. For many women, self-examination gives a sense of mastery over their bodies and helps to reduce anxiety. Those who do it sporadically – the BSE "dropouts" – say they forget, find it a hassle or are afraid of finding a lump.

The great advantage of BSE is in getting to know what the breasts normally feel like so that changes will be noticed. BSE sometimes picks up cancers that develop *between* routine mammographic or clinical screenings. And since many women don't get frequent enough medical checkups, BSE is a particularly valuable detection aid. It's an easily learned check, done once a month, in which women use their eyes and hands to detect breast changes. It *must* be done right, and it's best learned from a health professional.

Why Is BSE Training a Good Idea?

Very often BSE is incorrectly done, and it may even lead to a false sense of security, so that the wrongly done ritual stops a woman from getting adequate physician checkups. So it should be learned from a well-trained health professional who ensures that it's done right. One study found that even half an hour's BSE training greatly improved skill in detecting small cancers.

Although BSE hasn't been definitively shown to reduce the death toll from breast cancer, major studies under way will offer more conclusive evidence about its life-prolonging value. A joint study by the University of Toronto and the Mama Program in Helsinki has recently shown lower mortality from breast cancer in women who practice BSE than in non-practicers. The Toronto-Helsinki study followed a group of 29,000 Finnish women for the appearance of breast cancer. The results showed reduced mortality in those practicing BSE, regardless of age, presumably because they found cancers at an earlier, more treatable stage. Another recent study also showed mortality reduction in women who did BSE well.

How to Do BSE

BSE involves visual observation and probing all areas of the breast with the finger pads, applying pressure with a rotary movement. It is done regularly at the same time every month – preferably seven to ten days after the period ends. Post-menopausal women can do BSE on the first day of each calendar month. When they first try BSE many women complain that they find so many lumps and nodules in their breasts that they can't tell the difference between what's "normal" and what's "abnormal." The lumpiness should always be checked by a physician the first time it's felt, or if the woman is worried about it. The key is to distinguish any new lumps from the usual lumpiness, and the best way to learn what is normal for *you* is to become thoroughly familiar with your breasts. "It's amazing," says one woman, "how quickly and easily the fingertips come to recognize something new." Remember to *report any change* – gradual or sudden – to your family physician or other healthcare provider.

The Key Steps in BSE

Phase one: look for changes.

Stand naked about two feet in front of a mirror, with your hands at your sides, and examine the contours of each breast, searching for any asymmetry, distortion, swelling, unevenness, or redness. If you've always had differences in the size and shape of your breasts, these are normal for you.

Look for:
- asymmetry – any new difference between the two breasts;
- swelling;
- nipple discharge;
- skin scaliness, especially around the nipple;
- dimpling or puckering of the skin;
- persistent pink or red patches;
- retraction or inversion of the nipple.

With hands on hips, flex your shoulders forward and continue to look at the breasts and skin as above. Both breasts and nipples should react to the movement in the same way, with no skin dimpling or puckering. Lift your hands above your head and behind your ears and look again for the same changes.

If you notice a spontaneous discharge without squeezing the nipple, or if a discharge appears at another time of the month, consult a physician.

Phase two: Feel the breasts while standing.

Still standing in front of the mirror, feel each breast carefully with the finger pads with a probing, rotary motion to test if one area of the breast is lumpier than any other. Raise your left arm and use the pads of the fingers on your right hand to check your left breast and surrounding area, then reverse the

Breast Self-Examination – Phase One

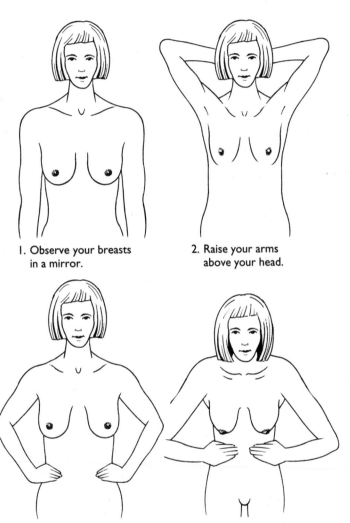

1. Observe your breasts in a mirror.

2. Raise your arms above your head.

3. Push your hands into your waist.

4. Push your shoulders forward.

process. Some lotion or powder may help your fingers glide more easily over the skin; some women like to do it when they're soaped up in the shower. Feel for any unusual swelling or lump under the skin. Some women use an up-and-down search pattern, others a rotary one. The crucial thing is to cover the entire breast. Check your armpit for lumps. Occasionally, the first sign of cancer is an enlarged node (gland) in the armpit. If a lump is found in this area, have a physician check it.

Phase three: Feel the breasts while lying on your back.
Stretch your right arm up and bend your elbow behind your head. Using the finger pads on your left hand, examine your right breast from the edge of the nipple in ever-larger circles out to the rim of the breast and then up toward the collarbone, shoulder and armpit. Move the fingers back and forth slightly to seek out irregularities. If you are full-breasted, be especially careful to probe thoroughly. Repeat on the other side.

Breast Self-Examination – Phase Two

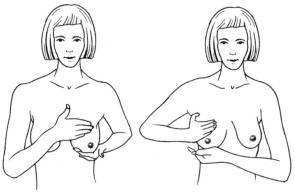

1. Cradle your left breast and gently feel it with the fingers of your right hand.

2. Cradle your right breast and repeat the palpation.

Breast Self-Examination – Phase Three

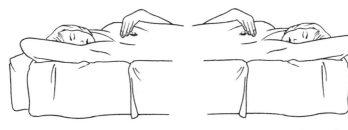

1. Lying down with your right hand behind your head, palpate your right breast with the fingers of your left hand.

2. Repeat this procedure with your left breast.

Never rush BSE. Even small-breasted women should allow a few minutes to examine each breast once a month.

Together with regular medical breast exams and mammography, breast self-examination can increase the chances of discovering breast cancer early. But note that *all three examinations* – BSE, clinical exams and mammograms – may be needed. While mammograms are the only way to spot tumors too small to be felt, they miss some cancers. Mammography can portray a normal breast even when a lump can clearly be felt – as happens quite often. So *never* let a negative mammogram rule out biopsy when BSE or a clinical exam finds a lump that arouses suspicion. Get a second opinion, or insist on biopsy, if you are worried.

Even if the mammogram is negative, suspicious lumps found by women themselves, or by clinical examination, usually need to be biopsied.

For more information about BSE contact your local cancer society or agency; as well, some drugstore chains and

In Praise of Breast Self-Examination

- BSE is simple to do once learned.
- It's easily learned from an expert.
- It's free.
- It's within your own control.
- It doesn't need any special equipment.
- It's not invasive.

pharmaceutical companies supply free information and shower cards depicting the steps in BSE. Consult the resource section at the back of the book for a list.

FIVE

What If a Lump Seems Suspicious?

If a woman discovers a new lump or thickening in one or both breasts, she should promptly report it to her family physician, or go to the nearest women's health clinic, breast center, breast-screening or diagnostic clinic, for advice and a thorough breast examination.

It's a good idea to take along a friend or relative as a "second set of ears" to help remember what was said, as women may be not only naturally anxious but also bombarded with lots of new information. Special tests may be suggested, for example a mammogram or ultrasound exam, and the woman may be referred to a surgeon and/or other breast specialists for further consultation.

If You Find a Lump – Don't Panic!

First and foremost, remember that a breast lump doesn't inevitably spell cancer. The majority of breast lumps biopsied are *not* cancer, but benign (noncancerous) changes. The best approach is cautious optimism until all the test results are in and there's a firm diagnosis. If it's benign women can stop worrying – and if it is cancer, they can start dealing with it.

Whom Do You Consult about Breast Lumps?

Family physicians, obstetrician-gynecologists or nurse practitioners are usually the first healthcare providers women consult about breast abnormalities. The family physician may refer the woman to a surgeon, breast specialist or breast clinic. "If the physician isn't very familiar with breast problems," counsels one breast expert, "request referral to a breast specialist." Nowadays there are many well-trained cancer specialists and breast diagnostic centers around, so try to find one nearby. Some cities and even smaller centers have breast-screening and/or breast diagnostic clinics or other specialist units that are a good place to start. Hospitals, medical schools and local health authorities can provide the names of breast clinics or staff physicians who specialize in breast problems. (See also the extensive resource guide at the end of this book.)

Deciding Whether a Lump Is Cancer

There's no way of knowing, just by feeling or touching it, whether a lump is cancer or some benign disorder, such as a harmless cyst. Physicians try to distinguish "definite" or distinct lumps from general breast nodularity. But deciding whether there is really a definite lump amid glandular breast tissue can be difficult. Benign masses (lumps) usually have smooth outlines and are mobile (not fixed but movable) – but not always. The only way to tell for sure is by further investigation with mammography, ultrasound and perhaps ultimately a biopsy to remove some tissue from the suspicious area and examine it under a microscope. (See chapters 8 and 9 for more on biopsies.)

Lack of pain is a characteristic but not dependable sign of cancer. Lumps that are hard and have indistinct borders *suggest* cancer, and so do those that are attached to the skin, but these are not reliable indicators.

Further Tests to Check Out Breast Lumps

If there is a lump, thickening or other breast abnormality, the next step is usually a mammogram and a visit to a breast surgeon to determine the need for biopsy. Slight delays in getting the tests or surgery done should not trigger blind panic. Even if it is cancer, the tumor has likely been silently growing for years, and a few days, even a few weeks, will probably make no difference to the outcome. If the suspicious area suggests a fluid-filled cyst, the physician may aspirate (drain) it in the office using a fine needle. Needle biopsy of a solid lump – removal of tissue samples for examination – can also be done. (See Chapter 8.)

Mammography May Provide Clues

Mammograms complement physical exams: some lumps that can't be felt show up on a mammogram, and some lumps felt by hand don't show up on the X-ray. Up to 15 percent of cancers felt by hand look normal on mammograms. The purpose of mammography is not only to characterize and precisely locate a lump, but also to find other occult (hidden) cancers that could be present in the breasts. Multiple cancers are not unusual, and simultaneous cancers in both breasts are reported in 3 percent of cases (as many as 65 percent of them are found by mammography alone).

If the combination of clinical exam and mammography does not provide enough information to tell whether a lump is cancerous, a biopsy is needed to take out some tissue from the suspicious area and examine it. Only a biopsy can confirm whether a lump is benign or malignant. In the past, when biopsy required open surgery, surgeons often hesitated to subject women to an operation in order to biopsy "gray area" lumps that were probably benign. But nowadays there are special biopsy techniques such as needle aspiration or core needle biopsy that can remove tissue samples without the need for surgery. (See Chapter 8.)

Never Reject Biopsy of a Suspicious Lump

"Do *not* rule out the need for further investigation and biopsy when there are any sinister findings, such as a clearly felt lump or asymmetrical breast change," counsels one Canadian cancer expert. "Never ignore a worrisome lump that you feel yourself, or one found by a physician, even if the mammogram is negative. Although in some instances the probability of a lump being cancer is vanishingly low, it is *never* zero. Any diagnostic method short of biopsy is only an educated guess."

To avoid missing a cancer, even if the physician says it's "nothing to worry about" and the mammogram seems clear, women should never ignore their own uneasiness about a lump.

The take-home message is that women should press for further tests, even if physicians downplay the risk, when they think there's something wrong. "If women feel something unusual," warns a renowned U.S. breast doctor, "get it biopsied, whatever the physician's opinion. Often a woman is sure she has a lump, the surgeon is sure she doesn't, and a year or two later a lump shows up on the mammogram." The woman may think the physician was careless. "But," continues the expert, "it is likely that the patient – who, after all, experiences her breasts from both inside and outside, while the doctor only experiences them from outside – *sensed* that something was amiss. If you are uneasy, seek another opinion. If you're wrong, it will put your mind at rest – if you're right, it may add some years to your life. A biopsy is minor surgery with low risks and potentially high gains."

Surgeons Explain What to Expect

In the old days, women were told before they underwent biopsy of a breast lump that, if the pathologist's quick examination of a frozen section showed signs of cancer in the breast tissue, they would have a mastectomy (breast removal) while still under the anesthetic as a "one-step" procedure. Nowadays, to ensure the most accurate interpretation and decide on the best treatment, women with breast lumps usually have a "two-step" procedure: first a biopsy to sample and test the abnormality for cancer; then, after a week or two – if it *is* cancer – surgery and other treatments.

"It is best to spell out the tests and treatment options ahead," says one surgeon, "as it reduces anxiety, demystifies the situation and lets a woman know what she could be in for. What I tell women for starters, if I'm not sure whether the lump is cancer, is that the lump must be biopsied, often by core [needle] biopsy without the need for surgery and hospital admission. If the worst comes to the worst and it *is* cancer, we'll then discuss the treatment options." Informing women accurately can reduce the fear of cancer, allows them to take part in the decision-making, increases their sense of control and decreases the sense of helplessness.

What Next?

If the biopsy shows cancer, the next step is surgery. Today's surgery for breast cancer is no longer necessarily *mastectomy* (total breast removal), but often just *lumpectomy* – removal of the lump and surrounding margins – along with some axillary (underarm) lymph nodes, to see if they carry signs of malignancy. "We do an axillary dissection to remove underarm nodes," says the surgeon, "as that's still our best guide to staging the cancer." Staging means establishing the extent and degree of the cancer in order to decide on the best type of therapy.

After surgery, according to the stage and extent of the cancer, most women also get some adjuvant (additional) therapy, either radiation, chemotherapy or hormonal treatment (or a combination), usually administered by an oncologist (cancer specialist).

Understanding what surgery and other therapy mean, what to expect, why, for how long and the likely side effects can help women adjust to the fact that they may have breast cancer. These days, women take an increasing part in the decision-making about their treatment and discuss options with the medical team.

Second Opinions?

Some women feel uneasy about the tests or treatment suggested, are not well enough informed or don't understand the choices. For them, a second opinion may be helpful. Dr. Susan Love of Harvard Medical School suggests in her book *Dr. Susan Love's Breast Book* that if women think they are belittling or insulting their physician by requesting a second opinion, they shouldn't feel that way. "It's your body and your life and you are seeking the most precise information possible in what could be a life-and-death situation. Most doctors will not be offended and if one is miffed don't be intimidated. Ask the family physician, surgeon or other specialist for a referral if you like."

SIX

Imaging the Breast

Breasts can be "imaged" by various means to reveal their inner structure and check for signs of cancer. Modern imaging methods include mammography (X-rays), sonography (ultrasound), CT scans ("slice by slice" X-ray pictures) and MRI (magnetic resonance imaging). Previously popular breast-imaging methods – such as *thermography* (heat-scanning) and *light-scanning* – have now been largely discarded.

Mammography

Mammograms remain today's most widely used and sensitive imaging tool for detecting breast cancer, even though they miss 10 to 15 percent of malignancies. The purpose of mammography is not only to evaluate a lump that's been discovered by the woman herself or her physician, but also to screen for abnormalities that are hidden and cannot be manually detected.

A mammogram is a special X-ray of the breast – "mammo" means breast and "gram" means picture. Mammograms look *into,* or "image," the breast's soft tissue, allowing radiologists to notice anything abnormal. Mammography can pick up very small nodules – about ½ cm (0.2 inch) across or even smaller – whereas lumps that can be felt by hand usually measure at least one cm (0.4 inch) in diameter. Mammograms can also detect tiny "microcalcifications" that are even smaller and can be warning signs of cancer.

Having a Mammogram
Doing a mammogram means squeezing the breast momentarily between two plates (one being the film-holder) to compress the tissue in order to get a clear X-ray picture. The entire procedure takes only a few minutes. Usually two views of each breast are taken. Special care is needed with women who have breast implants.

Having a Mammogram

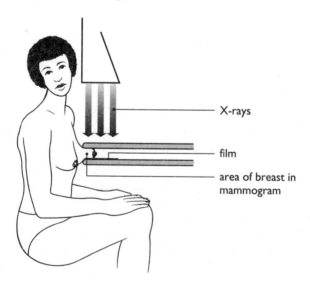

X-rays

film

area of breast in mammogram

While going for a mammogram may cause some apprehension, it should also bring reassurance that at least, if cancer is present, treatment can be speedily started. Some women find the compression needed to gain a clear X-ray picture uncomfortable, but most find it only mildly uncomfortable, and each X-ray takes only a few seconds. Apart from some transient pressure as the breasts are squeezed, having a mammogram isn't too distressing – lots of medical tests are worse! Some radiologists ask the patient to decide: "Can a little more pressure be applied for a better picture?" Many patients say, "Yes." The brief examination may save a breast or even a life.

How Do Mammograms Detect Cancer?

In an X-ray picture, benign breast lumps typically look uniform, rounded and smooth-edged, perhaps with a "halo" of surrounding fat. In contrast, cancerous lumps often have an irregular shape, perhaps with spicules or radiating strands; they look denser in the middle and may have speckled calcifications in or around them. To the expert radiologist's eye, such changes reveal or suggest the presence of cancer.

How Safe Is Mammography?

The equipment used in modern, well-run mammographic units has greatly reduced radiation dosages so that the risk from the amount of radiation is considered negligible. Modern X-ray machines deliver minuscule doses of X-rays, and the rays do *not* stay in the body.

By the time women reach the age where they're most vulnerable to breast cancer, they're also much less prone to radiation risks. With women below age 30, physicians worry about the hazards of radiation (because young breasts are more vulnerable to radiation damage and future malignancies), and hesitate to do mammograms unless really essential.

Getting the Best Mammogram

Since the quality of mammograms, the clarity of X-ray pictures and the ability of radiologists to read them varies widely, it's a good idea to have your mammogram at an up-to-date and reliable unit. The best are those dedicated to breast X-rays, ideally ones accredited by the Canadian Association of Radiologists or its U.S. equivalent. To make sure mammography conforms to stringent criteria, the American College of Radiology (ACR) began a voluntary accreditation program in 1987, and the Canadian Association of Radiologists (CAR) has done likewise. To earn either organization's "seal of approval," radiologists, their technologists and their equipment must maintain high standards of excellence, reviewed every three years. At present, CAR accreditation is voluntary, whereas in the U.S. accreditation is compulsory. If the hospital or X-ray unit isn't accredited, consider asking about the vintage of the equipment, whether it's used solely for mammography, the amount of radiation used for each picture and who reads the films. Radiologists who analyze breast X-rays to detect malignant changes require considerable skill and experience in spotting small deviations from normal. It takes an experienced eye to pick out small, diffuse or unusual cancers, especially in a dense or lean breast.

Mammography Has Its Limits

Mammograms show only those portions of the breast that can be compressed between X-ray plates. In breasts that are very glandular or dense, cancers may not show up against the normal breast tissue and may be hard to spot. But a similar tumor in the middle of fatty tissue will be more obvious. That's one reason why mammography is better at detecting cancer in the breasts of older women, in whom fat has replaced the glandular tissue.

While cancers typically have irregular margins and radiating strands, not all do. Although most cancers have recognizable features, some deceptively resemble benign cysts or fibroadenomas. When a woman has a "suspicious" lump, she can expect to have more than the routine two-view screening mammogram. The lump may be specially magnified to get a clearer image. Added X-ray views help to detect cancerous changes. Occasionally, cancers missed by X-rays are picked up on ultrasound (see below).

As yet, there's no standardized, agreed-upon way to express mammographic changes. While there's greater accuracy if

The Advantages of Mammography

- It's the best available early detection tool with which to detect breast cancer.
- It can spot very early and small cancers not felt manually.
- Mammograms can often detect breast cancers well before they're felt by physical examination.

The Disadvantages of Mammography

- It may give a "false positive" result suggesting that a harmless lump is cancerous, leading to needless anxiety and surgical biopsy. Some women have had several biopsies for benign lumps based on mammographic evidence. (However, the same holds true for physical breast examinations.)
- It isn't 100 percent foolproof and doesn't detect all breast cancers. Some cancers felt manually don't show up on the X-rays.
- There may be "false negatives" indicating no cancer when cancer is present, often because a cancer doesn't show up against a background of dense tissue, or because radiologists wrongly read or misinterpret the X-ray film.
- There is a theoretical small radiation hazard – depending on the dose and type of equipment used.
- The procedure can be briefly uncomfortable to some, and engender anxiety.
- It can give a false sense of security so that women ignore or neglect to report changes noticed between mammograms.

those doing or interpreting the mammograms also palpate (physically examine) the breast, it's a sobering fact that a seemingly "normal" mammogram provides no guarantee that a lump felt by hand isn't malignant, nor any absolute assurance that there is no cancer present. If a clinical exam, mammogram and ultrasound all indicate that a lump is benign, there's usually no cause for worry. But until the abnormal area is biopsied and the tissue is examined, there's no guarantee it's not malignant. The best rule is *"When in doubt, get a biopsy!"* (See Chapter 8 for more on biopsies.)

Ultrasound or Ultrasonography

Ultrasound has a smaller role than X-rays in imaging breast lumps and is *not* a screening test. It is used to determine whether a mass seen on the mammogram or felt by hand is likely to be a cyst or a solid lump. It is a *confirmatory* tool to see whether a lump is cystic or solid, as mammograms cannot show the difference. However, if ultrasound doesn't show a solid mass, there's no guarantee it's not there; it may simply not show up. Ultrasound is also useful for determining whether a breast implant has ruptured.

Ultrasonography is based on sonar – the apparatus used by the navy to "hear" echoes from submarines deep under water. Like submarines, tissues reflect sound waves (echoes) to a listening device that converts the echoes into electronic signals that appear on a screen or can be printed out as a "sonogram." Ultrasound *cannot* tell the difference between benign and malignant tumors. However, it is useful as a guidance tool for doing *needle biopsies,* to help the physician place the needle correctly.

Although mammography remains the chief breast-imaging method, ultrasound provides additional information. It is particularly useful in evaluating dense breasts that may hide

> **Uses of Breast Ultrasound:**
> • to differentiate cysts from solid masses;
> • to evaluate a lump not visible on the mammogram, especially in dense breasts;
> • to obtain additional information;
> • to guide procedures such as needle biopsies.

abnormalities, but it can also lead to needless investigation. In women under age 30, ultrasound may be the first imaging test done, as young breasts are sensitive to radiation and it is desirable to limit radiation exposure.

CT or CAT scans

Computerized axial tomography (CAT or CT scan) uses radiation to create cross-sectional pictures that give extremely detailed images. So far, they are not an effective way to examine breasts. The method employs more radiation than mammography, and sometimes requires the use of an intravenous material that can cause allergic reactions – possibly serious, even life-threatening.

Magnetic Resonance Imaging (MRI)

MRI creates images of the tissues and structures inside the body through a magnetic field without using radiation, but the process requires the patient to lie on a narrow table in a tunnel-like device within a powerful magnetic field, which can create intense anxiety in anyone who's claustrophobic. Within the walls of the tunnel, a special device measures how the body's hydrogen atoms react to the magnets. A computer converts the measurements to cross-sectional photo images, clearly showing the body's structure slice by slice. MRI is still in the early stages as a tool for diagnosing breast cancer. It's a cumbersome, expensive method, and cannot detect small telltale calcifications in the breast. Its ultimate usefulness in detecting breast cancer remains to be seen. It could become a valuable adjunct to mammography for examining suspicious lesions, and as a "staging" tool for breast cancer.

SEVEN

The Benefits of Breast Screening

Screening efforts and greater breast awareness have resulted in earlier detection of breast cancer than in previous decades, with greater promise of recovery. To date, we have three useful but imperfect screening tools for detecting breast cancer – breast self-examination (BSE), physical breast exams by a qualified health professional and mammography. None is foolproof in picking up cancer. BSE, clinical exams and mammography all miss some malignancies, but together they are our best way of finding breast cancer early. Screening mammography aims to detect "occult" (hidden) cancers lurking inside the breast.

The Great Screening Debate

The debate around mammographic breast screening focuses on the age at which it should begin, how often women should have mammograms and other issues such as the added value of breast self-examination. There is no longer any doubt that regular mammographic screening of women over age 50 reduces their death toll from breast cancer. The collected results of many studies conclusively show that mammographic screening of women aged 50 to 69 reduces death from the disease by about 30 percent. So screening is universally recommended for women in this age bracket. But the experts argue about the value of mammographic screening for women in their forties, since studies do not definitely show that it diminishes the death rate from breast cancer in that age group.

"Screening" Differs from Diagnostic Mammography
It's vital to distinguish screening from diagnostic mammography. Although the actual procedure is similar for both, their purpose differs.

Diagnostic mammography is used for women who already have some symptoms of breast abnormality, to help define the diagnosis. It usually takes more time than simple screening, as radiologists ensure that the suspicious area is in the X-ray field, or take extra "spot" or "magnification" views.

Screening mammography is used to detect unrecognized disease at an early stage in healthy women who have no symptoms or suspicions of breast cancer. It is a routine public health measure applied to large populations of women in order to detect hidden or latent disease so that it can be treated at an early stage, with the ultimate aim of saving lives. In other words, screening mammography is applied to asymptomatic women who have no known lumps, nipple discharge or other obvious signs, to detect small changes that may indicate cancer. Modern screening mammograms can detect cancers less than 0.5 cm (0.2 inches) in diameter, too small to be felt by hand. Since it is used on large numbers of healthy women, screening mammography requires careful assessment of its cost-effectiveness and benefits versus risks. In a world of finite health-care resources, the cost of saving one life by submitting thousands of women to mammographies must be carefully computed. Apart from the dollar costs, screening can lead to false-positive results, with needless biopsies and anxiety.

Screening Can Save Lives in the Over-50s

Six randomized, controlled trials of periodic mammographic screening in women aged 40 to 74 have all shown a reduction in deaths from breast cancer, especially in the over-50 age group, with a 20 to 30 percent reduction in breast cancer deaths among the screened, compared to unscreened, women. "The collected results of the trials," states one researcher, "convincingly show that regular mammographic screening reduces deaths from breast cancer in women over age 50, and that the cancers found by mammographic X-rays are consistently smaller than those discovered manually." Of tumors found by screening mammography, almost half are less than 2 cm in diameter (less than one inch) and unlikely to have spread. In general, the smaller the tumor, the better the outlook.

Why the "Magic Age" of 50?

There is no mysterious or fixed start-up age for the detection of breast cancer or the benefits of mammographic screening. It's just that most studies divide women into age brackets for research purposes, and to distinguish pre-menopausal and post-menopausal women. While research shows a conclusive benefit for screening women aged 50 and over, the benefit is inconclusive, or small at best, for women 40 to 49 years old. Therefore, while most health authorities support mammographic screening of women over 50, they argue about its benefits in younger women.

What About Mammographic Screening for Younger Women?

A few studies suggest benefits for screening women aged 40 to 49, but results depend on the follow-up time, and are uncertain and inconsistent to date. All but one study – the New York Health Insurance Plan, or HIP study – have so far shown little or no death-rate diminution from screening women under 50. After 18 years of follow-up, the HIP study found lower death rates from breast cancer for women screened under age 50. Swedish and U.K. trials have found negligible to modest benefits for screening women aged 40 to 49. The U.S. Breast Cancer Detection and Demonstration Project (BCDDP) claims some benefit for screening women under age 50, but the results have been contested.

Canada has conducted one of the largest-ever screening trials, the National Breast Screening Study, or NBSS. So far, the NBSS – like several other studies – has found no benefits for routine mammography in women under age 50. And those who conducted the study steadfastly reject the usefulness of mammographic screening for younger women. But others disagree. In general, outside the U.S., routine mammographic screening is restricted to women over 50. Some health agencies (mostly American) recommend regular mammograms for women in their forties, even though the studies have not conclusively proven that it reduces death rates from breast cancer. They argue that the 50-year dividing line is arbitrary and there is no compelling reason why early cancer detection shouldn't also benefit younger women. (In fact, many younger women request mammograms to put their minds at ease about lumpy breasts.)

Although most breast cancers occur in post-menopausal women, the disease also takes a considerable toll among women aged 35 to 50. About 20 percent of all breast cancer occurs in women under age 50; more than half the cases are detected by clinical examination, only about one-quarter more by mammography. This may be because X-rays are less efficient in finding cancer in the denser breasts of pre-menopausal women than in post-menopausal women, or because cancers grow faster in young women. In terms of life expectancy, younger women have even more to lose than the over-50s.

Those in favor of screening women aged 40 to 49 suggest it should be done annually as cancers tend to be more aggressive in younger women, and having mammograms every two years may result in some fast-growing interval cancers being missed. Women in high-risk brackets for breast cancer should ask caregivers about the benefits of having mammograms, and when to start.

Health authorities in various countries give different screening advice for women under age 50. The American Cancer Society, for instance, currently suggests that all women over age 20 do monthly BSE and have a clinical breast exam every three years up to age 40, then annually, and that all women aged 40 and up have a mammogram every one to two years. By contrast, the U.S. National Cancer Institute (NCI) shifted its former stance with the following statement in November 1993:

> There is general consensus among experts that the 1987 National Cancer Institute screening mammography recommendations, for women aged 50 and over [i.e., annual screening] be maintained. For women under age 50, the National Cancer Institute will provide a summary of existing evidence and data, and suggests these be discussed with each woman's physician or health care provider.

In Canada, each province has different screening recommendations. Only British Columbia and the Northwest Territories provide regular screening for the under-50s. The Canadian Cancer Society recommends breast cancer screening by BSE *for all women* by age 40, and mammograms every two years from age 50 to 69. Women at high risk for the disease should seek individual screening advice, and those who need screening under age 50 should be followed by a formal screening program, if possible. In Britain, only women over 50 are offered mammograms, and then only every three years.

Amid the conflicting medical opinions, how can women decide what's best for them, whether and when to request a mammogram and how often to have one? For women over 50 there's no question – regular mammograms are a good idea. But for a woman, say, in her late thirties, mid-forties or approaching age 50 the decision is more difficult. The best solution is to be as well informed as possible and make an individual risk assessment. Weigh up personal risk factors, taking into account family history, close relatives who have the disease, lifestyle, diet and other risk factors (listed in Chapter 11). If in a high-risk bracket, discuss the merits of mammography with the family physician, a specialist, or health professionals at a breast-screening center or diagnostic clinic. (See resource list at end of book.)

What's the Overall Canadian Screening Advice?

Most health authorities recommend mammographic screening for all women aged 50 and over, up to age 70 or beyond. In Canada, five provinces and one territory currently have programs that provide organized screening for women over 50, every two years or so. Besides regular mammograms, Ontario's breast-screening program also offers women clinical breast exams done by nurse practitioners and training in breast self-examination.

For Women Aged 50 and Over

Mammography is advised every two years. Alberta, Nova

Scotia, Manitoba, Ontario and Saskatchewan currently screen women aged 50 to 69 years or older, and Quebec also plans to screen women aged 50 to 69 years.

For Women Aged 40 to 49 Years
British Columbia offers routine mammographic screening to women aged 40 to 49. It is the only Canadian province that currently screens women under age 50 as part of an organized program.

For Women at High Risk of Breast Cancer
Mammographic screening may be advised under age 50, particularly for those known to be at above-average risk, such as women with mammographically dense breasts, those with atypical hyperplasia (found on biopsy), obese post-menopausal women and those with a genetic tendency to breast cancer (women whose mothers, sisters, grandmothers or daughters have or had breast cancer before menopause). "For women with a family history of the disease," states one Ontario breast-screening expert, "we recommend that screening start about five to ten years before the earliest breast cancer in the family."

American Breast Screening Guidelines
In the U.S. recommendations for breast cancer screening are complex and changing all the time. Currently, different cancer agencies suggest different screening guidelines. For example, the American Cancer Society no longer recommends a baseline mammogram before age 40 but does advise mammograms every one to two years for women aged 40 to 49, and every year after age 50. The American College of Radiology advises mammograms every year for all women aged 50 and over, as well as breast self-examination from age 20 onwards and an annual physical examination from age 40 on. The

National Cancer Institute (NCI) suggests annual mammographic screening for women aged 50 and over; for women under 50, the NCI advises that they discuss the need for mammograms with their healthcare providers.

Too Few Who Need It Go for Screening

Surprisingly, few of the over-50s who could benefit from X-ray screening seek or receive it. Notwithstanding widespread efforts to increase breast awareness, less than half the women aged 50 to 69 currently get breast screening. (In 1994, less than 40 percent of Canadian women over age 50 had ever had a mammogram.)

One reason why older women neglect getting mammograms may be the headlines describing screening arguments, or portraying breast cancer as a "young woman's disease." Many women avoid going for a mammogram, or delay consulting a physician about a lump, for fear of finding cancer. Cancer phobia – fear of "the big C" – is widespread and can prevent women from examining their breasts, getting medical attention or going for screening. Some women avoid mammography because they think that it will hurt or that X-rays are dangerous. Health professionals and activists alike are pressing for more uniform screening programs, and more education for women at risk.

EIGHT

Biopsies

Biopsy – the removal of tissue samples for examination under the microscope – remains the ultimate method for diagnosing cancer. Only a biopsy can confirm cancer. Breast biopsies remove tissue samples from the suspicious area, using a needle or surgical scalpel. If the lump is found to be cancerous, further surgery and other treatment may follow.

Formerly, biopsy samples were always removed from the breast by surgery, under general anesthetic. But modern image-guided, nonsurgical techniques that withdraw tissue samples with a needle are increasingly side-stepping the need for surgical biopsy. The newer methods are just as accurate but quicker, cheaper, less invasive and less nerve-racking, and require no general anesthetic. Since the majority of breast abnormalities investigated turn out to be benign, physicians prefer to avoid the discomfort and costs of surgical biopsy whenever possible.

Nonsurgical Breast Biopsies Ease Diagnosis

Nonsurgical biopsy methods can be done in the clinic or doctor's office or, if using "imaging" (X-ray or ultrasound) to guide the needle, in the hospital radiology (imaging) department. The methods include *fine-needle aspiration* – using a thin needle to withdraw fluid and some cells out of suspicious cysts – and the increasingly popular *large-core needle biopsies*, in which radiologists use a large-core needle to remove larger tissue samples, under X-ray or ultrasound guidance. This method is especially useful for small, nonpalpable (not felt by hand) abnormalities found by mammography or ultrasound. A needle biopsy is done as an "outpatient procedure." Following a short rest, the woman can usually carry on with her daily activities. Should the needle biopsy show the breast lump to be cancerous, surgery to remove the tumor and its surrounding "margins" (borders) will probably follow soon afterwards.

When it confirms the presence of cancer, needle biopsy avoids the need for two bouts of surgery in short order, one to withdraw and examine the tissue samples, the second to complete tumor and underarm node removal. It's bad enough to face having cancer, without having to do so while recovering from surgery and a general anesthetic. Without the weakness and post-operative grogginess that usually follow a general anesthetic, women can make major decisions about cancer treatment in a more clear-headed manner.

Pathologists Examine Biopsy Specimens

The breast tissue removed during biopsy is microscopically examined by a pathologist, a physician who specializes in detecting the cellular and tissue changes that accompany disease. The tissue to be examined is either frozen for immediate or "quick" analysis, or embedded in paraffin for slicing and a more thorough and accurate examination of the entire sample. A full pathology report takes three to ten days to prepare.

The larger the tissue samples, the easier it is for pathologists to detect signs of cancer. If there are just a few cells for cytological examination, as often happens with fine-needle aspiration, an abnormality may be missed. Larger tissue samples, such as those obtained by large-core needle or surgical biopsy, allow pathologists to do a thorough *histological* examination (looking not just at cells but at the total tissue architecture). Given enough tissue, skilled pathologists can determine the type and stage of cancer present, whether it is still localized or invasive, aggressive or slow-growing, and indicate the "prognostic factors" that predict outlook and help in planning treatment.

Fine-Needle Aspiration Biopsy (FNAB or FNA)

For this procedure the woman sits or lies on her back. The skin around the lump is swabbed with antiseptic. A fine, hollow needle is inserted into the abnormal area or lump to withdraw

Current Breast Biopsy Options

- *Fine-needle aspiration* – FNA or FNAB (fine-needle aspiration biopsy) – takes only a few minutes to withdraw cells from the suspicious area for cytological examination (of single cells). If the abnormality or lump can be felt, FNA is done in the physician's office; if not, it is performed under ultrasound guidance in the hospital imaging or radiology department.
- *Large-core needle biopsy,* done by a radiologist in the imaging department, using a large-core needle in a spring-loaded device, uses *stereotactic* (X-ray) or ultrasound guidance to remove "cores" or plugs of tissue from the suspicious area for histological examination.
- *Open or "formal" (surgical) biopsy,* the traditional surgical method, is done with or without fine-wire X-ray localization to pinpoint the area to be sampled.

any fluid present (and also some cells), to be sent for evaluation to detect signs of cancer. If the lump can't be felt manually, then ultrasound or, less commonly, mammographic guidance is used to place the needle in the right spot. The whole procedure takes just a few minutes and there is minimal discomfort.

If the lump is a fluid-filled cyst, needle aspiration may turn out to be the treatment as well as the means of diagnosis. Once the fluid is withdrawn, the cyst collapses and the lump may vanish. If part of the lump remains after drainage, further tissue sampling – by core or surgical biopsy – will follow, as

Fine-Needle Aspiration

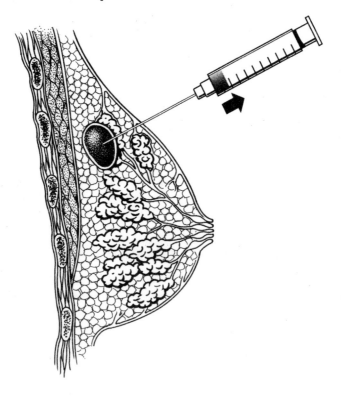

there could be a cancer lurking beneath or around the cyst.

If the lump being tested is a solid mass, the physician may hold it between the fingers and push the fine needle back and forth to free some cells and suck them into the syringe. The cells withdrawn are smeared onto a glass slide or put into alcohol and then sent to the pathologist. It normally takes about a week to get the pathology results. If the FNA result shows definite signs of cancer, there's often no need for more tissue sampling; the next step is surgery. However, if the FNA biopsy result on the cells withdrawn is negative, there's no guarantee that cancer isn't present so a core or surgical biopsy must follow to rule out malignancy.

Fine-needle aspiration of solid lumps has many drawbacks and is rarely diagnostic of cancer. In almost 30 percent of cases it obtains no or too few cells for analysis. Even when single cells are obtained, pathologists need specialized expertise to analyze them rather than whole tissue slices. Moreover, if the result is uncertain the needle may have penetrated a benign area in or around a cancer, so although the pathologist finds "no malignant changes," the result requires further investigation. A cancerous lump may contain both normal and malignant cells, and if the needle withdraws benign rather than cancerous cells the "no cancer" result is false. If the FNA result is inconclusive and the report states "too few cells for evaluation," a surgical or core biopsy will usually still be needed, especially if there is a strong suspicion of cancer. Fine-needle aspirations miss up to one-third of cancers later identified by core or surgical biopsies, so many clinicians prefer other biopsy methods.

In general the three biopsy methods complement each other – FNA may give a quick answer confirming cancer, but if it's negative or inconclusive a core or surgical biopsy is needed to give a definite answer.

The Main Advantages of FNA:

- done easily and painlessly in the doctor's office or hospital imaging department;
- provides an instant cure when cysts are completely drained;
- doesn't involve surgery;
- may identify cancer quickly, skipping the need for surgical tissue sampling.

The Main Disadvantages of FNA:

- can only "harvest" a few cells, not large clumps of tissue. About 30 percent of pathologists' reports on FNA samples return saying: "Not enough tissue" (for examination).
- cannot distinguish localized, non-invasive from invasive cancer;
- gives uncertain answers, as the needle often misses cancerous areas; even multiple fine-needle passes may entirely miss a cancer, in which case FNA becomes a needless and anxiety-arousing step.

Large-Core Needle Biopsies

Large-core needle biopsy overcomes many failings of FNA and is increasingly popular. Core biopsies are done in the clinic or hospital imaging (radiology) department, under ultrasound or mammographic guidance. Using large-core, 14-gauge needles, several cores of tissue are removed for examination, under light freezing.

Imaging devices (X-rays or ultrasound) automatically guide the core-biopsy needle to the suspicious area. A spring-loaded device or "gun" is used to insert the biopsy needle into the breast, quickly removing cores of tissue – about the size of rice grains – from the target area. Several samples – usually five – are taken from the site, to reduce the risk of "false negatives." If X-ray (stereotactic) guidance is used, the woman usually lies face down, but in some cases she sits. With ultrasound as the guidance tool, she lies on her back during the procedure and the radiologist guides the needle by watching a monitor.

Afterwards, the woman uses an ice pack for a few minutes to stop bruising. Acetaminophen is taken to reduce pain if needed (not ASA as it increases bleeding). Normal activities can often be resumed the same day, but no very strenuous activities should be attempted for a week or so.

Core biopsies are as accurate as surgical biopsies, but quicker, simpler, cheaper, less disfiguring and less traumatic. In the hands of radiologists skilled in imaging techniques, the accuracy of core biopsy approaches that of traditional surgical biopsy, revealing both the type of cancer and its invasiveness.

During an X-ray-guided core biopsy, the woman lies face down on a special table, her breast protruding through an opening. This position prevents fainting, which can happen if

Having a Core Biopsy

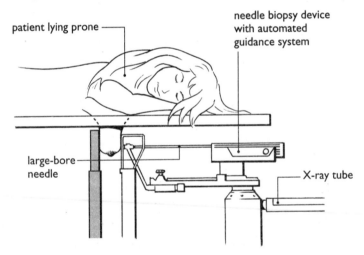

Whether ultrasound or X-ray imaging is chosen for core biopsies depends on the type of abnormality, which imaging method provides the clearest picture and the equipment available. Some lesions (for example, those in very dense breasts) are better imaged with ultrasound, while others show up better with X-rays. If both ultrasound and X-rays give equally good images, ultrasound is often the preferred guidance tool.

women sit during the procedure and become anxious. The radiologist works out of sight, under the table, and digital computers calculate the exact location of the abnormality. The area to be examined is "frozen" and a tiny nick is made in the skin for entry of the needle. The breast is compressed to permit accurate imaging. Once the needle is in place, the automated device makes a small noise as it is inserted. Core-needle biopsy is not painful. Most women say that it doesn't hurt or that there's no more discomfort than having one's ears pierced. The main dis-

The Main Advantages of Core Biopsy:

- as accurate as surgical biopsy but cheaper, quicker, non-invasive and less psychologically traumatic;
- avoids the need for general anesthesia, producing less postoperative grogginess;
- gives less scarring than surgical biopsy, therefore does not hinder future mammographic interpretations;
- does not have many failings of FNA (insufficient specimens, false-negative results and need for expert cytopathologists);
- permits full tissue work-up;
- can identify malignant or benign abnormalities such as fibroadenoma, hyperplasia (tissue overgrowth) or hyperplasia with atypia (a possible warning sign for future breast cancer). The cores of tissue are usually sufficient to type the cancer, showing whether it's invasive or localized and providing information about its grade, hormone receptors and other prognostic factors that predict outcomes;
- eliminates the need for two surgical procedures: one for diagnosis, the second for treatment. Once diagnosis is established by core-needle biopsy, the woman and her caregivers can discuss the surgical and follow-up treatment.

The Main Disadvantages of Core Biopsy:

- samples are still quite small – if no cancer is found, surgical biopsy may still be needed; when the core biopsy and mammographic results differ, surgical biopsy is often recommended;
- core biopsy units are not yet widely available;
- the technique is not suitable for lumps very close to the nipple, near the chest wall, in the armpit or close to the skin surface.

comfort is some neck stiffness from lying on the stomach for half an hour or so. (A few units use a sitting position.)

If the result is "no cancer," the core-needle biopsy has avoided the need for surgery. Women understandably feel immensely relieved if it shows a benign condition without the trauma and anxiety of a surgical operation. However, with some benign conditions (such as atypical ductal hyperplasia), surgical biopsy may still be advised to rule out concerns about early cancerous changes. Women in whom the core biopsy result is negative are advised to return for a repeat mammogram six months later to be sure nothing has changed. Although core biopsy lacks most disadvantages of FNA and is as accurate as surgical biopsy, it cannot be used in certain situations, such as a very deep breast lesion in a very small, thin breast (too little tissue), or for those unable to lie face down comfortably for the required time (for instance, women with severe arthritis or other medical conditions).

Open Surgical Biopsy

Surgical biopsies are either *excisional* – completely removing the lump – or *incisional,* removing just a piece for examination.

Excisional biopsy is used for small breast lumps that can be felt by hand. If the lump turns out to be malignant, further surgery may be required to remove the rim or margins of tissue around the tumor, to make sure the entire cancerous part is eliminated and also to remove some underarm lymph nodes for detection of malignancy and to determine the stage (extent and invasiveness) of the tumor.

Incisional biopsies are now only occasionally done – for example, in the case of a very large lump. "We try not to remove too much," explains one surgeon, "because if it's benign – as it is in most cases – we don't want to leave a large scar or disfigure the breast."

Surgical biopsies are usually performed in hospital as "same-day" procedures, or in outpatient clinics. The operation may be done under local or general anesthetic, depending on the extent of surgery needed and the surgeon's and woman's preference. The type of anesthesia – as well as the type of biopsy – is determined by the size and location of the abnormality.

For lumps that are small, well defined and near the breast surface, the surgeon may use local anesthesia, injected near the surgery site. (Local anesthesia may also be used after the incision is closed, to lessen postoperative discomfort.) General anesthesia will be used for larger excisions.

A quick "frozen" section or on-the-spot analysis is sometimes done in an area adjoining the operating room while the woman remains anesthetized on the operating table. The pathologist quickly "freezes," slices, stains and examines a sliver of the breast tissue under a microscope. If the pathologist is 100 percent sure the sample is cancerous, it gives an immediate answer and enables the surgeon to take operating decisions. But frozen sections often give false-negative results. Confirmed diagnosis must still await the full pathology report. Cancer cannot be ruled out on the basis of a negative frozen-section result. Only the complete, detailed analysis of the entire tissue sample and its margins from edge to edge – by a "permanent" method, embedding the tissue in paraffin wax, slicing it and examining it bit by bit – can rule out or confirm cancer.

After the biopsy operation and a few hours' rest, the woman can usually go home, accompanied by a relative or friend (people often feel groggy after general anesthesia).

Fine-Wire Localization Aids Surgical Biopsy
The sophistication of modern mammography alerts clinicians to the presence of abnormalities or lumps too small to be felt. For such small lesions, an excisional biopsy is often done with

Open Surgical Biopsy

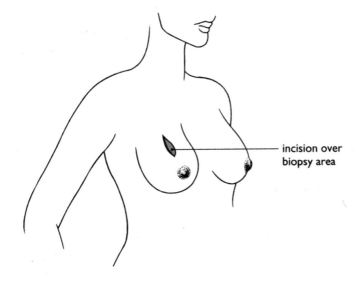

incision over
biopsy area

the help of *fine-wire localization*, a technique in which the radiologist pinpoints the exact area to be biopsied. Fine-wire localization is especially useful when mammography reveals the presence of tiny *microcalcifications*, scattered specks of calcium that may indicate early breast cancer. Microcalcifications rarely herald cancer unless clustered in one area of the breast, but are usually investigated by biopsy.

In fine-wire localization, the woman is taken to the radiology department just before surgery. She sits positioned as if for a mammogram and, under X-ray or ultrasound guidance, the radiologist inserts a needle into the breast with its tip near the abnormality. Through the needle the radiologist then feeds in a very fine wire – no thicker than a hair – with a tiny hook at its end that fixes it in place to mark the suspicious spot for the surgeon.

The wire stays securely anchored by the hook until the

surgery, when it is removed together with the biopsy tissue. The piece removed is X-rayed again while the patient is still on the operating table to be sure the surgeon has indeed taken out the suspicious tissue. (In some centers, dye is injected into the suspicious spot and used to guide the surgeon.)

Many women have several biopsies over a lifetime, without any of them finding malignancy. Having several biopsies does *not* increase the likelihood of developing cancer later on. Nonetheless, a biopsy finding of "atypical" hyperplasia (atypical breast cells), which occurs in about 4 percent of benign breast biopsies, *does* portend greater risk, and the condition must be carefully monitored (see Chapter 2). And even after a negative biopsy, women over 50 need to continue with regular breast screening as they remain at high risk of developing breast cancer.

Awaiting the Biopsy Report

The complete pathology report can take a week or more to prepare – a wait that can seem interminable – but the full report is crucial for deciding the best treatment. It's a period that takes considerable patience and requires much sympathy and support for the woman awaiting the results. A diagnosis of any cancer evokes chilling anxiety. But a diagnosis of breast cancer delivers a double blow to women. Not only does it signal the presence of a potentially lethal disease, but it also strikes at a woman's self-image, sense of femininity and sex appeal. Women deserve all the attention and understanding they can get at this time.

NINE

The Pathologist's Report

The pathological examination of the tissue samples obtained by biopsy confirms the diagnosis of breast cancer, and establishes the size, type and characteristics of the tumor. The pathologist examines the margins surrounding the tumor, as well as any axillary (underarm) lymph nodes removed, for signs of cancer. According to the tumor's characteristics, the prognosis – probable outlook – is also assessed. "Cancer is not an alien from outer space," notes one renowned oncologist, "and with all the focus on new tumor markers and fancy prognostic factors, we tend to forget that the woman's own resistance and immune system play a role in the outcome and survival."

The cancer is typed and graded according to the pathologist's detailed evaluation of the tumor and the state of the underarm lymph nodes – whether they are "positive" (showing the presence of cancer) or "negative" (cancer-free). The pathologist's analysis and report on all the factors assessed helps clinicians plan the treatment. Some women have very slowly progressing forms of breast cancer that have been quietly growing for years without producing symptoms, and that, once removed, do not recur. Others have fast-growing, aggressive tumors that have already spread when discovered. Breast cancers in younger women (under age 40) tend to be more aggressive than those in older women.

Cancers accompanied by "positive" underarm lymph nodes that also show signs of cancer have a worse prognosis, with higher chances of recurrence, than "negative" cases where the nodes show no malignancy. This is because the presence of cancer in the underarm nodes suggests that cancer cells may already have spread from the breast to other sites. Removal of the underarm nodes does not influence survival; it just helps to stage the tumor and predict the likely outcome. Treatment is geared to the state of the underarm nodes, the cancer's biological features or "markers" and the woman's age.

The Pathologist's Examination

The tissue samples that arrive at the pathological laboratory are embedded in paraffin wax, specially stained and thinly sliced for examination under the microscope. Any underarm nodes removed are also examined for signs of cancer. The *histological* examination looks at both the overall tissue architecture and individual cells. (If only a few isolated cells are supplied – as happens with a nipple discharge or fine-needle aspiration – a special *cytological* examination of individual cells must be done.)

The examination covers the entire tissue sample and reveals whether the cancer is large or small, localized or invasive, fast- or slow-growing, aggressive or mild, and whether or not it has hormone (estrogen and progesterone) receptors. Taken together, all the "prognostic" factors predict the cancer's behavior. The final pathology report becomes part of the woman's medical file and is used to select and track therapy.

Any extra preserved tissue is carefully stored so that it can be re-examined in future if questions or problems arise.

The pathology report usually has three sections: the gross (as seen with the naked eye) observations, the microscopic description and the summary or final diagnosis. The report describes the tumor's size and whether it was all successfully removed – shown by "clear" margins with no remaining signs of cancer. Experts stress the need for wide margins and removal of plenty of tissue rather than too little. "It is usually possible to remove wide, safe margins," notes one surgeon, "without distorting the breast too much, still leaving it acceptably attractive." Better a wide excision than increased chances of cancer recurrence.

No Magic Markers, But Telltale Features
Besides lymph node status, the prognosis or outlook for breast cancer is determined by the tumor's biological features. Molecular tumor factors play an increasing role in helping oncologists estimate the probable chances of recurrence, and the likely efficacy of different therapies. While no one tumor characteristic is a magic clue to its behavior, an ever-increasing number of biological markers are being discovered that help physicians decide on the best postoperative therapy.

The shades of abnormality seen under the microscope reveal a range of changes from benign to strongly cancerous. For example, the cancer cells may be so distorted and *undifferentiated* (featureless) that they no longer resemble breast cells. Greatly altered or undifferentiated cancer cells that have lost their unique breast characteristics suggest an aggressive cancer and a worse outlook than those with better-differentiated cells that remain more "breastlike." *Nuclear grade* (the appearance, size and density of the cell nucleus) is useful for assessing the outcome of breast cancer. The higher the grade, the worse the outlook. Another telltale feature of an aggressive cancer is vascular and lymphatic *infiltration*, when cancer cells are seen in the lymph system or blood vessels.

Cells that respond to female hormones contain specialized receptors into which the hormone molecules fit (like a lock and key) to stimulate growth. The growth of breast cancer cells that possess hormone receptors may be accelerated by female hormones such as estrogen and progesterone. Breast cancers high in estrogen or progesterone receptors are generally less aggressive and more "breastlike," and are likelier to respond well to anti-estrogen therapy (with tamoxifen or removal of the ovaries) than those low in these receptors.

Other biological tumor factors that may indicate tumor aggressivity include "ploidy" – chromosome numbers; various growth factors (for example, cathepsin-D – an enzyme indicating high tumor aggressivity); and "S-phase" – the number of cells seen in the process of dividing and replicating (copying) their DNA content. The tumor's biological markers are especially useful in helping to determine the best therapy for node-negative cases.

The right treatment for women with no cancerous nodes is still much debated. About 70 percent of women with node-negative breast cancer do very well with tumor removal only, while the other 30 percent are at risk of relapse and need additional postsurgical therapy. "The problem," says one breast specialist, "is to decide which of the lymph-node-negative cases will do well and need no extra treatment, versus those likely to do badly who need additional treatment. Perhaps some of the new tumor markers will help us select which node-negative cases are at greater risk."

However, as one pathologist notes, "the plethora of new biological markers and prognostic factors coming on board, and their rapid commercialization, can be confusing, as there is a lack of standardization among different laboratories in measuring them and deciding the cut-off points for what's considered high or low risk. There is a need to standardize laboratory techniques and reporting methods."

In assessing the prognosis, physicians consider the chances of local cancer recurrence on the operated side, the probable years of "disease-free" survival and the possibility of distant spread, which determines the likely *overall survival time* (years) after diagnosis. The reduced risk of relapse or prolongation of life achieved by various treatments can be expressed in absolute terms as "number of recurrences," actual "years of survival" or as a percentage or proportion.

"Small" Does Not Necessarily Mean "Early"

While, in general, the larger the cancer, the greater the risk that it has already metastasized (spread), a small cancer does *not* guarantee local confinement. Broadly speaking, stage 1 to stage 2 breast cancer is still confined to the breast and potentially curable, "low-risk" cancer. Stage 3 is "advanced" breast cancer that has infiltrated the skin and muscle or other structures, and stage 4 is metastatic cancer that has spread to other parts of the body. (For ways to stage breast cancer, see chapters 12 and 13.)

Most oncologists believe that breast cancer survival is linked not just to tumor size and type but also to predetermined genetic features and to the cancer's potential for metastasis. Even under the best of circumstances, it's not always possible to detect cancer before it spreads. Although delays in diagnosis are popularly blamed for decreased survival prospects, the detection of breast cancer is often impossible until many years after the first cancer cell appears in the breast, by which time it has divided many times and a few cells may already have escaped and lodged elsewhere. Thus the outcome depends as

Features That Influence Survival Prospects:

- *age* – some younger women have a worse outlook than those over age 50;
- *underarm lymph node status* – chances of disease-free, long-term survival are best when no underarm lymph nodes are cancerous, and progressively worse the greater the number of nodes found to harbor malignancy;
- *tumor size* – the smaller the diameter, the better the woman's chances. Tumors under one cm (0.4 inches) across have a low recurrence rate. Relapse risks rise with increasing tumor size;
- *tumor invasiveness* – in-situ (localized) cancers have not "invaded" or penetrated beyond the breast; invasive ones have;
- *infiltration* of the blood or lymphatic system;
- *nuclear grade and differentiation* – the appearance, size and density of the cell nucleus;
- *necrosis* (presence of dead and dying cells) in the tumor – a sign of rapid cancer growth, which outstrips the nutrient supply from the blood;
- *high "S-phase"* (high rate of proliferation/multiplication) – which indicates the number of actively dividing tumor cells;
- *DNA ploidy* – chromosome number and DNA variations (abnormal chromosomes);
- *absence of certain "neu-oncogenes"* (genes involved in the spread of cancer) – which suggests disordered, unhalted tumor growth;
- *specific "growth factors"* that stimulate growth – such as cathepsin-D, linked to tumor aggressivity;
- *estrogen/progesterone receptors* – receptors in breast cancer cells where female hormones can bind and stimulate cancer growth.

much on the *biology* of the tumor as on its size, or even more. Although many women survive longer if diagnosed at an early stage, this does not necessarily mean that their lives are prolonged; it may just mean that they are aware of having the disease sooner. (See also Chapter 10.)

Reactions to the Diagnosis of Cancer

Given the media blitz about breast cancer in recent years, most of us living in North America are aware that it's a common disease that can strike any woman. But for the individual who learns she has been diagnosed with breast cancer, the news is a shock. The immediate reaction is usually cold, debilitating fear, anxiety about surgery and possible disfigurement, about the loss of femininity and sex appeal, uncertainty and apprehension about treatments and the disruption of life. Hearing the diagnosis is the first major hurdle and source of distress. Later periods of particular stress and anguish are undergoing the often lengthy treatments and the first recurrence.

Many women feel helpless, don't know what to expect or how they'll cope; they may feel buffeted by the impersonal, mechanized workings of the medical system and confused by the different answers they're given by various caregivers. Nonetheless, some women don't appear particularly distressed about mortality at the moment of discovering they have cancer. They may be more upset about possible surgical disfigurement, the uncertainty and the hassle of treatments. Only later – often after therapy ends – does the full impact of the news really hit them.

TEN

Breast Cancer Overview

A couple of decades ago hardly anyone mentioned breast cancer except in hushed undertones. Today it is a frequent front-page media story. Activist groups have sprung up to politicize the disease and push for greater understanding, better treatment and more research funds. Entire art shows are devoted to the subject. This chapter outlines some salient facts about the disease.

Putting the Numbers in Perspective

Heart disease, stroke and lung cancer each kill more women in Canada and the U.S. than breast cancer. Heart disease kills more women than *all* cancers combined. One in three people eventually gets cancer and one in four will die of the disease. The three most common types of malignancy among women in North America are breast, lung and colorectal (bowel) cancer. In the U.S. and Canada, breast cancer is the most common cancer among women, but lung cancer is the leading cause of cancer deaths in both women and men; it's responsible for one-fifth of all cancer deaths in women and one-third of all cancer deaths in men. In Canada, about 17,000 women a year are diagnosed with breast cancer and 5,400 die of it (compared with 5,800 female deaths a year from lung cancer and 10,000 from heart disease).

Cancer statistics are reported among a given population or number of people – "per 1,000," say, or "per 10,000." *Incidence* is the number of new cases reported each year, *prevalence* is the number of cases at any given time and *mortality* is the number of deaths attributable to the disease per year.

Many people claim that there has been a dramatic rise in breast cancer incidence among young women. In fact, the increase has been in women aged 55 and older. Since cancers are now detected at an earlier stage due to mammographic screening and better surveillance, part of the rise may be due to earlier detection. Examining the numbers, we see that U.S. and Canadian survey data show a rise of about 30 percent in the annual incidence of breast cancer from 1980 to 1987, and a continued rise up to 1989, then a levelling off, and since 1991 a slight downward trend. The steep rise in incidence coincided with the rise in mammographic screening, and the discovery of smaller and more localized cancers – so cancers are probably just being found sooner. Since the effect of this earlier detection has now settled down, the apparent surge in incidence has started to level off. Survival may also be improving slightly; in 1993, overall five-year survival was 78 percent, compared to 64 percent in the 1960s. Studies show a slight recent decline (3 to 6 percent) in mortality, which some attribute to a combination of screening and better treatment.

Analyzing the "1 in 10" Statistic

One of the scariest statistics being publicized is the fact that "one in ten women will get breast cancer." But this is a *lifetime* risk that only applies to women when they get older, over

Chances of Breast Cancer at Various Ages among Canadian Women	
Age	Risk
30	1 in 2,472
40	1 in 262
50	1 in 63
60	1 in 28
70	1 in 14
80	1 in 12
85	1 in 10
From Health Canada (1994)	

age 85; it does not apply in younger age groups. The risk of a woman in her 30s or 40s developing breast cancer is far lower than it is for older women. A 40-year-old woman has one chance in 63 of developing breast cancer by age 50, one chance in 28 by age 60 and one chance in 14 by age 70. Even a woman of 75 has not reached the one in 10 figure. It doesn't pertain until she is around age 85 or 90. Since cancer usually develops very slowly in the elderly, most of these women will die of something else long before breast cancer claims them. Curiously, although women of 65 are far more likely than 40-year-olds to get breast cancer, they seem less aware of their susceptibility and less watchful for signs of the disease than younger women.

Incidence Varies with Race and Family History
Above 40 to 45 years of age, white women have the highest breast cancer rates, followed in order by blacks, Hispanics and Asians. Jewish women are at above-average risk, while Mormon and Seventh-Day Adventists are at lower than usual risk. Incidence rates in the northern U.S. tend to be higher than those in the south, and rates in urban areas are slightly higher than those in rural areas. Never-married women and those who are childless are at higher risk than married women

or those who have borne several offspring. Women of high socioeconomic status are at greater risk. A recent study from Finland found that women in the highest occupational and educational brackets had breast cancer rates twice those in lower socioeconomic brackets or less well paying jobs. These differences probably reflect variations in childbearing patterns and age at birth of first child.

Variations Give Clues to Causes
The variation in breast cancer rates among different races and in different countries, together with studies in migrants, gives clues about possible causes. Environmental factors are thought to play a key part in breast cancer. International differences in breast cancer incidence are attributed to variations in body weight, diet and reproductive factors – age of menarche (onset of menstruation), age of first childbirth and number of children borne. Studies suggest that Japanese women may have lower estradiol (estrogen) levels than North American women, possibly due to diet or less body fat, which may explain their traditionally lower breast cancer rates. But more research is needed to clarify the picture.

A very early menarche, under age 12 – an increasing trend in North America – increases the chance of developing breast cancer, as does having a child at an older age, another increasing trend in the West. Other suspected causes of breast cancer include a high-fat diet, being tall, being overweight (post-menopausally) and lack of exercise at a young age – before and during adolescence.

What Is Breast Cancer?
Breast cancer covers a wide spectrum of disease in which some tumors are aggressive and metastasize quickly, while others develop slowly, perhaps taking decades to show symptoms.

Breast Cancer:
Some Key Facts and Figures

- *Breast cancer is a chronic, potentially fatal disease of varying type and severity,* ranging from tiny changes or microcalcifications detectable only by X-ray to large, palpable tumors that may be invasive and may have spread to other areas. A breast cancer can grow quite large without causing any pain or other symptoms.
- *Breast cancer occurs more often in the left breast than in the right* (perhaps because the left tends to be larger and has more tissue), and in about one percent of cases primary tumors are found in both breasts at the time of first diagnosis.
- *In North America breast cancer will affect one woman in ten* who reaches 85 or more years, and is second to lung cancer as a cause of cancer deaths in women. At present about 17,000 women a year are diagnosed with breast cancer, and 5,400 die of it.
- *Most breast cancers occur in women over age 50.* The older the woman, the greater the risk.
- *Many breast cancers are still discovered by women themselves,* the average size at discovery being two cm.
- *Finding a cancerous breast lump early* – especially at a stage when it's too small to be felt but is detectable by mammography – can improve survival time.
- *Breast cancers removed when less than one cm across,* with no cancer cells found in the underarm lymph nodes, give excellent survival chances.
- *Mammographic screening in women over age 50 can reduce the death toll from breast cancer* by up to 30 percent. But mammography misses about 10 to 15 percent of cancers, and up to 40 percent of cancers in the dense breasts of young women.
- *The best way to check for breast cancer* is to get regular physical examinations by a competent healthcare professional, practice well-taught BSE (breast self-examination) and have mammograms every two years after age 50.
- *Men get it too* – about one percent of all breast cancers in North America occur in men, with an incidence around 1 per 1,000.

Cancer usually begins as a clump of abnormal cells, at first confined to a small area, later perhaps infiltrating nearby tissues. A few cancer cells may escape from the original or "primary" tumor and spread to distant parts of the body to form *metastases* (secondary cancers). Breast cancer can remain localized or "in-situ," or become invasive. Some breast cancers rapidly penetrate nearby tissues and spread – sometimes within months, especially in young women – while others take 10, 20 or more years to become invasive, and some never spread. Breast cancers can occur in the breast's milk ducts or in its lobes.

Very Early In-Situ Cancers and Their Significance

Modern mammography can detect very early breast abnormalities at a pre-invasive or precancerous stage, identifying dormant cells that are likely to develop into cancer five, ten or more years down the road. These appear as tiny calcifications that may become invasive cancers if left alone, but if they are removed in time the cancer may never develop.

The early changes are termed *carcinoma in situ* ("in place" and not invading nearby tissues). They can remain dormant for long periods, even for the woman's lifetime. Ductal cancer in situ, or DCIS – within the breast's ducts – is far more common (80 to 90 percent of in-situ cancers) than lobular cancer in situ, or LCIS, within the breast's lobes. The progress of these in-situ cancers varies according to their type and biological make-up, and whether they arise in lobular or ductal tissue. In-situ cancers are localized and rarely form a lump that can be felt or cause any pain. They pose a treatment dilemma as many, left alone, either never progress or grow very slowly. Yet, left untreated, they can become invasive – usually over a period of years – occasionally in just a few months.

In the "minimal breast cancer" category most experts include:

- ductal carcinoma in situ (considered cancerous);
- lobular carcinoma in situ (considered by most not to be cancerous but a marker for future cancer development);
- microscopic microcalcifications.

Ductal carcinoma in situ (DCIS) is far more common than LCIS and becomes invasive cancer in a quarter of those in whom it occurs. Post-mortem studies of women who died from other causes often reveal the presence of unrecognized DCIS that never gave any trouble. The development of DCIS occurs under hormonal influences; cells pile up in the breast ducts rather like rust in a pipe. This is intraductal *hyperplasia* or "overabundance of ductal cells." After a time, the excess cells may begin to look peculiar or *atypical;* later they may come to resemble cancer, and·this is when they are termed *intraductal carcinoma in situ,* or "cancer confined to the duct." On a mammogram, DCIS often appears as a cluster of calcification. Although the condition may never progress beyond this stage, there's always a chance that it will become invasive, so the abnormal patch is best removed.

Lobular carcinoma in situ (LCIS), often found around the time of menopause, accounts for only 5 to 10 percent of all in-situ cancers. Not a distinct lump, LCIS is more of a thickening, widely scattered through breast tissue. It's considered a "marker" for cancer and cannot easily be removed without taking off one (or even both) breasts, as the risk affects both sides equally. In one famous study, out of 211 patients with lobular cancer in situ, only 17 percent (36 women) developed invasive cancer over 30 years, suggesting that LCIS is a "risk factor" for cancer but not cancer itself. LCIS is usually only discovered when a biopsy is done to evaluate another lump or breast abnormality. The treatment options are to monitor the breast regularly with mammograms, or to remove both breasts. Such a sledge-hammer approach may seem drastic in an era when larger cancers are often managed with lesser surgery. But the risk of subsequent cancer for those with LCIS is lifelong. (See Chapter 12 for more on DCIS and LCIS.)

Minimal micro-invasive cancer less than one cm (0.4 inches) in size has a favorable outlook and may be treated by breast or lump removal. The term "invasive" means that the cancer has already invaded nearby tissues. A breast cancer of one cm has usually been growing for several years before detection. Even a 0.5 cm tumor, barely detectable on a mammogram, has already doubled its cell numbers many times, and scientists know that metastasis (spread) can occur within the first 20 cell doublings of a breast tumor. In general the risk of spread is less for small tumors, and studies suggest excellent survival rates in node-negative women after removal of tumors measuring less than one cm. (However, invasive tumors less than one cm still have a recurrence rate of 28 percent unless the breast is irradiated after lump removal.) Local recurrence rates are less after mastectomy.

Since tumor cells divide more rapidly than normal cells, they need extra oxygen and nutrients to support their rapid growth, and new blood vessels may develop to bring them the needed nourishment – explaining why tumor "vascularization" is a bad prognostic sign, even for small cancers.

New Concepts of Breast Cancer

Today's view regards breast cancer as a potentially *systemic* disease almost from its start, which can affect the whole body from an early stage and must be treated accordingly. Therapy therefore focuses primarily on halting or abolishing distant spread. Regular checkups by the oncologist or breast surgeon – checking for cancer in the second breast and for possible recurrences – are a lifelong necessity for all who have had breast cancer. In fact, through the regular and frequent follow-up medical visits, many women develop a long-standing relationship with their cancer physician and may come to regard him or her as a primary caregiver.

A Psychologically and Emotionally Searing Disease

Breast cancer is a disease that delivers a double blow to women. It not only arouses anxiety about treatment and fear of death, but also strikes at the very heart of a woman's self-image, femininity and sex role. It can profoundly affect her sexual and social relationships, and also undermine her self-confidence as a woman. The psychosocial effects can be profound and far-reaching but, thanks largely to awareness-raising efforts of activist and survivor groups, the medical fraternity is beginning to recognize the emotional, psychological and social impact of breast cancer and take it into account when offering treatment. Today's women are generally better informed about the disease, more aware of their options and more involved in the decision-making about therapy.

Looking Ahead – Possible Advances in Therapy

Breast cancer mortality has remained almost steady for half a century, despite efforts to discover more effective therapy or

What Starts Cancer Off?

Current theory suggests that cancer results from cumulative mutations (changes) in the genes that regulate cell growth, so that cells grow out of control and form the cancer. Cancer arises mainly through changes (defects) in the RER or *replication error repair* genes that normally repair damage to the cell's *deoxyribonucleic* acid, or DNA, as fast as it occurs. Flawed RER genes can't pick out and correct the molecular DNA errors, which can pile up (imagine a faulty spell-check in a word-processing program). Then, each time the DNA replicates at cell division, the error is also copied. A fault in the RER genes can also destabilize nearby genes, leading to abnormal cell division and cancer.

Generally speaking, the body's immune system recognizes cancer cells as abnormal, and destroys them. But sometimes the immune system cannot cope and cancer wins the day. Any method that can effectively bolster the immune system may help fight cancer, and much research is directed along these lines.

a true preventive method. A breakthrough or "magic bullet" is unlikely, as cancer is too complex. Progress will more likely depend on a broad-based attack on many fronts. "Toxic cell kill," notes one leading oncologist, "is not the ultimate answer. What's needed is *not* ever more potent cancer-killing agents, but finding some way to reverse the malignant process, perhaps by anti-tumor growth factors that turn off tumor growth, or gene therapy to block the action of cancer-causing genes." These solutions may be some way off, but meanwhile there are a few advances on the horizon.

Boosting the body's defense mechanisms to tip the balance toward destruction of cancer cells is one strategy. Biologically based "immunotherapies" such as lymphokine-activated killer (LAK) cells and heat shock proteins (recently produced by genetic engineering) may stop tumors developing. But the work is only preliminary.

Preventing cancers from vascularizing – capturing a blood supply – with agents such as "growth factor inhibitors" is another method being investigated. Once tumors manage to acquire a blood supply, their growth can increase a thousand-fold, so blocking the growth factors that allow this to occur could make cancers shrivel and die. Vascularization also permits cells to escape into the bloodstream and create metastases elsewhere in the body. Blocking the vascularization can help to prevent this spread.

New biological tumor markers now being uncovered, such as growth factor receptors or genetic markers, will reveal more about the nature of an individual tumor and allow better tailoring of therapy.

Understanding how mutations or damage to the oncogenes (cancer-related genes) and other portions of DNA force cells to behave abnormally and become cancers might explain why secondary breast tumors occur in some tissues, such as liver and bone marrow, but almost never in others, such as muscles, and could lead to drugs or gene therapy that turn tumor cells back to normal, or at least inactivate them.

Advances in bone-marrow and stem (blood-forming) cell transplants offer promise.

Inhibitors for secondary tumors are another avenue being explored. Recent research reveals that primary tumors sometimes stop dormant secondaries elsewhere in the body from growing, but that once the primary is removed by surgery, the inhibition disappears and the secondary tumor rapidly expands. If the factor that inhibits the secondary tumor growth could be identified, we might be able to manufacture it. Research into this possibility is progressing apace.

A drug called gestodene is a component in some newer types of combined contraceptive pills; preliminary evidence suggests that it may help to prevent breast cancer. Other drugs being investigated include vorazole and liarazole, which affect hormone receptors in the tumor and may stall its growth.

Innovative tests are being developed to help identify breast cancer patients who might benefit most from chemo- or hormone therapy, such as *DNA flow cytometry*, and new *oncogene* measurements.

Use of a synthetic hormone, somatostatin, is being tried to halt tumor growth.

Chemoprevention – therapy with tamoxifen and the hormone *human chorionic gonadotropin* – may prevent cancer in women at above-average risk and is being investigated.

Support groups, survivor networks, self-help groups, counselling and education are becoming crucial aspects of battling the disease.

Breast Cancer Activism Raises Awareness
During the past decade, vibrant breast cancer "survivor" and

activist movements have sprung up in North America, Britain and elsewhere, dedicated to fostering awareness, informing women about the disease, developing truly "informed consent," improving treatment and raising research funds. Breast cancer support networks and activists have made enormous inroads in improving the management of breast cancer, making women more aware of their options, empowering them to make better choices, giving them a greater sense of control and helping them cope better with the disease – improving the quality of life for many.

Dr. Susan Love, a U.S. breast surgeon, was one of the first to raise awareness about and politicize breast cancer. Following on her heels, many women have bravely spoken out about their plight, lifted the veil of silence, revealed the painful reality, paraded their mastectomy scars and hairless heads after chemotherapy – to get breast cancer out of the closet and bring concerned people together to discuss the issues.

The survivor alliances and activist organizations can give women the information and support they seek. Their ultimate aim is to help those with breast cancer make rational choices about their treatment in partnership with the medical team. As opposed to the high-tech medical approach, with its quantitative, interventionist methods, the breast cancer movement adopts a more "woman-centered," holistic, low-tech approach that fosters a sense of control, promotes non-toxic treatments and, above all, looks for prevention.

The activists use various awareness-raising tactics, such as the 1993 cover of the *New York Times Magazine* portraying a bare-chested woman displaying her mastectomy scar. Other activities include organizing self-help groups, preparing pamphlets and holding meetings. Once women manage to move beyond the despair and grief of having cancer, some find that helping others in the same plight and joining advocacy groups helps them fight the disease.

Artists Take Up the Cause

Artists and poets are now using their talents to demonstrate sympathy for the sufferers and survivors of breast cancer. In 1993 the Washington National Museum of Women in the Arts ran a 14-painting exhibit by artist Hollis Sigler, herself a breast-cancer survivor. In Britain in 1995, London's Barbican art gallery had a large exhibition of paintings and drawings by Susan Macfarlane, portraying intimate scenes of women in various stages of breast cancer treatment and recovery, aiming to demystify clinical practice. The paintings convey deep compassion. One, for instance, depicts a young woman on the day after surgery learning arm exercises; another symbolizes meditation. The Woodlawn Arts Foundation recently funded a cross-Canada art tour called "Survivors in Search of a Voice," which opened at Toronto's Royal Ontario Museum, displaying the work of 24 artists. Their works depicted the randomness and erratic nature of the disease, the problems of battling it and the harsh technology of today's medical care.

ELEVEN

Who's Most at Risk?

Canada and the U.S. are world leaders in breast cancer rates, which are also particularly high in countries such as Denmark, The Netherlands and Hungary, and far lower in other countries such as Thailand, China, Japan, Africa and Algeria. Epidemiologists believe the variation has to do with lifestyle and environmental influences and also with reproductive factors such as age of menarche (onset of menstruation) and childbearing patterns. But risk factors apply to groups or populations; estimating one's own individual risk is more difficult.

Weighing Up Your Risks

Breast cancer is not restricted to those at high risk. Anyone can get it. The overall risks depend on biological features over which women have no control – such as increasing age, genes (hereditary characteristics), mammographic breast density (as seen on an X-ray), levels of female hormones (estrogens) in the body – and lifestyle factors that can be modified, such as diet (amount of fat eaten), alcohol intake, exercise level and age of bearing children.

In weighing up your risks for breast cancer, consider both family background and non-heritable factors. Most breast cancers are not inherited but *sporadic*, triggered by multiple environmental "hits" that damage the genetic material, DNA. Identified risk factors for breast cancer include being tall, post-menopausal obesity, high breast density, a diet rich in fat and low in fruit and vegetables, excess alcohol consumption, insufficient vigorous exercise (especially at a young age), and exposure to estrogens and possibly some environmental agents such as organochlorides in DDT and other pesticides – although this link remains unconfirmed.

Women with several close family members who had breast cancer – especially at an early age, and particularly in both breasts – may have inherited a predisposition to breast cancer and be at above-average risk (in some cases men as well as women). However, only about 4 to 5 percent of all breast cancer is hereditary. In other families, several members may get the disease because of shared environmental or lifestyle factors.

Exploring the Genetic Connection
Having one or more first-degree relatives (mothers, sisters, daughters, grandmothers) who had breast cancer doubles the risk. If *both* the mother and a sister or grandmother had breast cancer, the risk is especially high, particularly if the cancer was diagnosed at an early age before menopause, and if it affected both breasts. Members of such cancer-prone families may carry a "cancer-susceptibility" gene that gives them a high probability of getting the disease. (A gene is a segment of one of the DNA molecules within our chromosomes – inside each body cell – that determine our genetic make-up.)

Recent research has discovered two mutant (altered) genes that confer susceptibility to breast cancer – BRCA1, on chro-

A Breast Cancer Susceptibility Gene

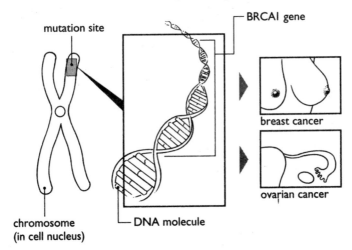

mosome 17 (blamed for about half the inherited breast cancer cases), and, more recently, BRCA2, on chromosome 13. These genes affect only a few families, accounting for about 5 percent of all breast cancers. The mutant genes are likely but *not certain* to cause breast cancer at some future date, perhaps decades later.

The BRCA1 gene is inherited in a so-called "autosomal dominant fashion," meaning that it's passed on from one parent to 50 percent of the offspring, or that *half the children of an affected parent* are likely to inherit it. But it's only an "average" risk, and in any one family all, none or some of the children may inherit the altered gene. Moreover, those who carry the cancer-susceptibility gene are not *certain* to get the disease. They have about a 90 percent chance of developing breast cancer during their lifetimes, and a 50 percent chance of developing it by age 50 – or a 10 percent chance of *not* getting it at all. The gene is not the cancer. Individuals born with the faulty gene will only develop cancer if other cancer-causing "hits" occur during their lifetimes.

Although people with the mutant BRCA1 gene have a high chance of developing breast cancer (and possibly also ovarian cancer), these cancers will only develop later in life, so carriers may not know for years or even decades whether they're in the 10 percent who won't get the inheritable cancer, or among the unlucky ones who will. If a woman with a strong family history of breast cancer reaches the age of 65 unaffected, she probably didn't inherit the predisposition.

Many BRCA1 carriers are also at risk of ovarian and colon cancer, although cancers of the ovary and colon (bowel) tend to develop later than those in the breast. In contrast, the BRCA2 mutant gene doesn't elevate ovarian cancer risks but puts male relatives at risk for breast cancer. (Men can transmit the breast cancer susceptibility genes to their daughters or sons.)

Genetic tests can now identify people who carry mutant BRCA1 or BRCA2 genes, so carriers can watch for early signs of the disease and get it treated promptly, or maybe take preventive action. But at present, testing for these genes is offered only on a research basis to a few cancer-prone families. In the not too distant future, however, the tests may become widely available, and could open a "Pandora's box" of potential problems with many ethical, social and psychological implications. Both the genetic information and the uses that will be made of it are now being discussed, and are in a process of transition.

Those found to carry cancer-susceptibility genes may feel stigmatized and labeled as "ill," even though they have no symptoms and may never develop the cancer. They may face job and insurance discrimination. (Insurance companies and employers could obtain and use genetic information to blackmark people, denying them benefits or employment.) Those who test negative may experience "survivor guilt" for not carrying the dreaded gene. Family feuds sometimes arise between members who want to be tested and those who don't. Genetic counseling before and after the tests is essential to help people understand the tests and recognize the implications.

What are the choices for a woman carrying a BRCA cancer-susceptibility gene? She can simply have frequent medical checkups to catch the earliest sign of breast (or ovarian) cancer, and get appropriate treatment. Or she can opt for bilateral mastectomy to remove both breasts *before* they develop cancer. (Perhaps she should also consider surgery to remove the ovaries.) But these are drastic considerations for people likely, but not certain, to develop cancer, especially as neither operation is 100 percent foolproof. Even after preventive bilateral mastectomy, there's a small chance of developing cancer in the chest wall (or in the abdomen after ovary removal). In future other preventive strategies, such as gene therapy, may prove more effective.

Take the case of Sarah, aged 27, whose mother and older sister had breast cancer when young (before age 40) and who has a teenage sister. (Her grandmother died of breast cancer before Sarah was born.) Clearly, with three close relatives who developed breast cancer at a young age, Sarah's at high risk, with a 50 percent chance of having inherited it from her mother. She decides to get advice at the local genetic clinic. The counselor suggests a test to look for the mutant genes. She's told ahead that even if she does not carry these genes, there's still the usual chance of getting *sporadic* cancer. The test is positive. Sarah does carry the BRCA1 gene. She decides to have bilateral mastectomy – removal of both breasts – even though there's no sign of cancer as yet. The genetic counselor explains that even if she has both breasts removed, there's still a small chance of developing cancer in the chest wall, and of getting ovarian cancer later on, but that she could be among the 10 percent of BRCA1 carriers who would *never* develop breast cancer.

Sarah is also informed that the body-image change due to bilateral mastectomy can be hard to face, and that she may want to consider breast reconstruction. As well, she's told that a double mastectomy will *not* alter the risks to her children, who could still inherit the BRCA1 gene. Sarah is also advised to consider telling her younger sister about the gene, so that she too can think about having the test.

These are tough questions. Should Sarah tell her younger sister, and warn more distant family members, that she has tested positive for the cancer-susceptibility gene? What about her employers? Would she be at a disadvantage in the job market if people knew she carried a gene for a potentially deadly disease? What are the legal implications? To deal with such dilemmas, members of "high-risk" cancer families who consider genetic testing need detailed pre- and post-test counseling to make sure they can handle the possibility of carrying a cancer-susceptibility gene. Some people from cancer-prone families refuse genetic testing or deny the danger, and sometimes, rather than seeking extra care, they shun the necessary surveillance, perhaps even failing to get advice for any breast lumps they find.

Cancer in One Breast Means Extra Risk in the Other

A woman who has cancer in one breast has two to four times the average risk of a primary cancer in the opposite breast, particularly if she's young when the first cancer appears, or has a family history of breast cancer.

Weight and Height Are Risk Factors

Tallness is associated with a modest elevation in breast cancer risk and most studies find that a heavy body weight and obesity increase the risks of breast cancer in post-menopausal women, although obesity seems to be protective in pre-menopausal women. The increased risk for obese post-menopausal women may stem from their higher estrogen levels, as estrogens are produced in fat tissue by conversion from other molecules.

Mammographically Dense Breasts More at Risk

A recent Canadian study is one of several that have shown that women with mammographically dense breasts have about six times more chance of getting breast cancer than those with "loose" (fattier) breasts. The high breast density cannot be determined by "feel" but only shows up on mammograms; it can occur as often in pendulous or "floppy" breasts as in firm, hard ones. Researchers speculate that the dense breast tissue may contain extra-abundant growth factors that stimulate cancer formation. Dense breasts are more likely to be found in women who start to menstruate young than in those who start their periods later. Breast density also seems to be increased by exposure to estrogens, leanness and alcohol consumption (which also increases the body's estrogen levels).

Estrogen Plays a Key Role

There's clear evidence that ovarian hormones such as estrogen and progesterone play a key part in breast cancer development, probably by increasing cell division. (The prime role of estrogen in the body is to promote growth of tissues related to reproduction, including breast tissue.)

Lifetime exposure to estrogen significantly influences breast cancer growth – the more the estrogen exposure, the greater the risk. Women who have had their ovaries removed before age 35 have greatly reduced rates of breast cancer. Women with an early menopause – whether natural or due to ovary removal – also have a lower chance of developing breast cancer. Women who start to menstruate before age 12 have a higher risk, because of extra years of exposure to estrogen. (Breast cancer risks are tripled in women who start to menstruate at age 10.) This may explain why women who delay childbearing or have no or few children have a higher risk: they are exposed to estrogen for a longer time. Pregnancy shuts off estrogen production. In addition, in women who breastfeed, lactation halts ovulation, stops periods and curtails estrogen production for as long as it continues, so prolonged periods of breastfeeding may reduce the risk. A delayed menopause prolongs estrogen exposure and increases breast cancer risks.

Experts speculate that some of the apparent increase in breast cancer may be due to long-term use of estrogen-containing oral contraceptives. Amid the morass of conflicting results, a recent British study showed a slightly elevated risk of breast cancer in young women on the pill, and more recent U.S. studies also showed a risk for those taking it for ten or more years. However, the World Health Organization currently reports no increased risk for breast cancer from taking the contraceptive pill. No change in current contraceptive strategies is advised, but the possibility needs to be closely monitored; substantial numbers of women have taken these hormones for many years.

Menopausal hormone therapy with estrogen (usually with added progestin) is also thought to slightly increase risks of breast cancer. Adding the second hormone, progestin – a form of progesterone – was thought to offset the risk, but recent evidence suggests that the progestin is not necessarily protective against breast cancer. The scant information available to date suggests that the risk for women using both estrogen and progestin for hormone therapy is at least as high as, and possibly higher than, that for women using estrogen alone. One large Swedish study showed an increased risk of breast cancer in women receiving estrogens alone and a possibly greater risk in those taking progestins. U.S. research also suggests that long-term estrogen treatment, starting during or after menopause, may elevate breast cancer risks. The current evidence adds up to a possible but unconfirmed elevation in breast

Hormone Replacement Therapy after Breast Cancer: Yes or No?

With women living longer, and undiminished rates of breast cancer, the question arises as to whether or not women who had breast cancer before menopause should take hormone replacement therapy (HRT) to offset menopausal discomforts. Women are being diagnosed at an earlier stage with breast cancer; some undergo early menopause from the treatments, and with long life-expectancies, and low risks of breast cancer recurrence, some may wish to go on HRT.

Most medical experts strongly discourage HRT for women who have had breast cancer, but attitudes are changing as women express concerns about the risks of osteoporosis (bone fragility) and heart disease, not to speak of hot flashes and other menopausal distress. They are wondering whether it might be possible to go on hormone therapy, at least for a few years. A report from the U.S. Centers for Disease Control evaluated the proportional increase in risk of breast cancer for each year of estrogen use. The risk did not appear to increase until after at least five or six years. Among women with a family history of breast cancer, those who had *ever* used estrogen-replacement therapy had a significantly higher risk than those who had not.

"Women who have had breast cancer or are at high risk should be wary of estrogen therapy," counsels one University of Toronto expert. He warns women and their medical caregivers "*not* to ignore the possibly increased risk of breast cancer from estrogen therapy." But this modest risk must be balanced against the probable benefits of hormone therapy – reduced chances of heart attack, lowered risk of osteoporosis and relief of menopausal discomforts. Together with their physicians, women should consider the pros and cons of post-menopausal estrogens.

cancer risks in women who take post-menopausal hormones for six or more years.

Diet and Breast Cancer

Diets high in calories and rich in animal fats seem to increase risks of breast cancer; those low in fat and high in fruit and vegetables (five to ten servings a day) seem to decrease risks. Recent evidence suggests that phytoestrogens in soya products, and olive oil, may reduce breast cancer risks, although the precise diet–breast cancer link remains unclear. High-fat diets are known to promote breast and bowel cancer in animals, but some researchers blame excess calories rather than too much fat for the elevated cancer rates. In any case, eating less fat, in particular saturated fat, is a generally healthy plan, and if fat consumption is reduced it not only benefits the cardiovascular system but can also reduce cyclic breast pain in those who suffer from it. (See also Chapter 20.)

Drinking Alcohol May Increase the Risk

Drinking moderate to low amounts of alcohol (one drink a day, or less) slightly elevates breast cancer risks, possibly because alcohol raises estrogen levels. A large meta-analysis (pooling results from many studies) shows a wide variation in the link between drinking and breast cancer, but it's worrisome enough to give women reason to watch their alcohol intake. "Women are in a double bind," notes one expert. "While moderate drinking (one to two drinks a day, but *not* every day) seems to protect the heart, it might raise breast cancer risks."

Lack of Exercise When Young Is Another Risk Factor

Recent studies have linked breast cancer to a lack of vigorous exercise when young, particularly before puberty and during adolescence. Parents should encourage their daughters to engage in sport and other vigorous activity from a young age onwards as a protective strategy against breast cancer – and as a general health measure.

Summing Up the Risk Factors

Unmodifiable risk factors:

- increasing age – being over age 50, the greatest risk factor;
- family history, affecting 4 to 5 percent of those who get breast cancer – people who carry the newly discovered BRCA1 or BRCA2 genes are liable to get cancer at an early age and may also be at increased risk of colon, ovarian and prostate cancer (in men);
- country of birth (race);
- early menarche – starting to menstruate before age 12 – because of extra years of estrogen exposure;
- late menopause (after age 50) – giving extra years of estrogen exposure;
- certain benign breast conditions such as atypical hyperplasia (tissue hyperactivity, with atypical cells), multiple papillomas and very large cysts;
- high breast density (as seen on a mammogram);
- cancer in situ – either lobular carcinoma in situ (LCIS) or ductal carcinoma in situ (DCIS).

Modifiable risk factors:

- never having borne children;
- few or late pregnancies (first full-term pregnancy after age 30 to 35); the greater the number of ovulatory cycles before the first pregnancy, the greater the likelihood of getting breast cancer. Women with first pregnancies before age 25 have a reduced risk;
- regular alcohol consumption – more than four to six glasses of wine a week or its equivalent in liquor or beer;

How the Different Risk Factors Compare

Strong (risk over 4 times normal)	Moderate (risk 2 to 4 times normal)	Weak (risk 1 to 2 times normal)
• previous cancer in one breast • family history of pre-menopausal breast cancer, especially if in both breasts • past breast biopsy showing hyperplasia with atypical cells • mammographically high breast density	• over 30 years old at birth of first child • past breast biopsy showing atypical hyperplasia • post-menopausal obesity	• first menstrual period before age 12 • menopause after age 50 • history of post-menopausal breast cancer in close relatives • female hormone use for more than 10–15 years, for either contraception or hormone replacement • moderate to heavy alcohol use • diet rich in animal fat (possibly)

- post-menopausal obesity – linked to a slight increase in breast cancer risks (but pre-menopausally, leanness seems to increase risks).
- prolonged use of estrogen-containing birth control pills, especially before a first full-term pregnancy – this may slightly increase risk, although the studies are inconsistent. The new low-dose pills are not thought to confer extra risk unless started very young and taken for more than seven to ten years continuously;
- hormone replacement therapy (HRT) – the link between post-menopausal estrogens and breast cancer remains unclear, but the evidence adds up to a probable but uncon-

firmed rise in risks among those on HRT for several years;
- radiation (exposure to environmental X-rays) – especially in very young women (under age 30), although diagnostic X-rays (used medically) do not increase risk;
- lack of vigorous physical exercise at a young age, especially before puberty and during adolescence;
- miscellaneous risks such as electromagnetic fields, organochloride residues, silicone breast implants, smoking and abortions – implicated but not proven to increase chances of developing breast cancer.

Note: Despite this list, most breast cancers appear in women with none of these known risk factors (other than age). *All women are at risk.*

TWELVE

Breast Cancer Management

In deciding on the most effective therapy for breast cancer, clinicians consider both the risks of *local* recurrence on the operated side and chances of *distant* spread. A thorough discussion with the medical team will determine the best type of surgery and postoperative therapy. There is no universally accepted method or agreement among medical experts about the "best way" to treat the thousands of women who develop breast cancer each year. Despite the vast sums spent on cancer research, there has been no major breakthrough in treatment, although some women are cured by current methods. Today, most women get some form of adjuvant (additional) treatment after surgical tumor removal to eradicate any lingering cancer cells and improve survival chances.

Today's Multi-Specialty Management
After surgery to remove the cancer, women are now generally referred to specialists for further advice and treatment, perhaps at a specialized cancer center or clinic. They can expect to be cared for by a team of healthcare professionals including the

Overall Management of Breast Cancer:

- *diagnostic biopsy* (to sample and analyze the abnormal tissue, testing it for cancer);
- *treatment, which includes:*
  - *local control* – surgery (lumpectomy or mastectomy) to remove the tumor and also some underarm lymph nodes to be tested for cancer;
  - *radiation to the operated side* after lumpectomy – to stop local recurrences or tumor progression;
  - *systemic (whole-body) control* – to destroy cancer cells that may have escaped beyond the breast, using chemotherapy, hormonal treatment or both.

Usual Steps in Breast Cancer Treatment

Diagnostic biopsy
Pathologist's report
Surgery to remove tumor and nodes; pathological examination
Staging the cancer: by nodal status, tumor characteristics and presence or absence of distant disease
Adjuvant systemic therapy

Local: radiation after lumpectomy to prevent recurrences	*Systemic:* hormonal therapy or chemotherapy to destroy cancer cells that may have escaped the breast (or both)

family physician, breast screening and diagnostic specialists, radiologists, pathologists, surgeons, nurses, counselors, physiotherapists, psychologists and, in particular, oncologists (cancer specialists). The treatment approach is based largely on the pooled results of many clinical trials that examined survival rates around the world following different kinds of surgery and various postoperative treatments. Careful analysis of the collected results of many studies, in the so-called "Oxford Overview" (showing improved survival), has led to today's treatment strategy, which is continually being updated as the results of long-term trials come in.

The *radiation oncologist* administers radiation therapy and the *medical oncologist* usually plans and supervises postsurgical drug and hormone therapy. Additional (adjuvant) therapy will be geared to the woman's age – whether she's premenopausal or post-menopausal – and the tumor's stage and characteristics. Since treatment strategies vary from center to center, women should seek advice from the most knowledgeable, up-to-date clinic and breast specialists around and, above all, from ones they trust and feel comfortable with. If they are not satisfied that they are getting the best possible, most current treatment or obtaining the information they seek, a second opinion may be worthwhile. They can request a referral to a specialist for consultation by asking their family physician or other caregiver.

Gentler "Two-Step" Strategy
When the biopsy and pathological report show the presence of cancer, surgery is usually the next step, to excise the malignant tumor and some axillary (underarm) lymph nodes to be tested for cancer. In many cases, the diagnosis and subsequent surgery for breast cancer are now done in two stages. First, the lump or abnormal tissue is biopsied to see whether it's cancerous, then the treatment options are discussed and the chosen surgery and subsequent therapy carried out. Delaying treatment by a few days or a week or two does *not* endanger the woman or worsen the outcome. The two-step process gives women time to think over and discuss options with the medical team. However, in certain instances the two-step rule doesn't apply; for instance, if a needle biopsy confirms the presence of cancer, only one operation is required to remove the tumor and some axillary nodes.

The modern method is gentler than in the old days, when a woman with a suspicious breast lump was told that the abnormal area would be cut out while she remained on the operating table, and quickly scanned for signs of malignancy with a frozen section, and that, if cancer was found, the breast would be removed while she was still under anesthetic. She would then awaken with her whole breast gone. This drastic procedure, done in one fell swoop, meant that a woman was "put under" not knowing whether she'd come out of the anesthetic with a small biopsy scar or with her entire breast gone.

Lumpectomy or "Lump Only" Removal Is Becoming Standard

If the cancer is small and confined to the breast, with no sign of distant spread – as it is in over 70 per cent of cases these days – surgeons usually suggest "conservative" surgery (lumpectomy) to excise the cancerous lump and surrounding margins (edges) but not the whole breast, usually also removing some underarm nodes to be tested for cancer. Lumpectomy is gradually replacing mastectomy for small cancers. It's becoming more popular not only for cosmetic reasons but also because most of the breast cancers discovered today are smaller (under 4 cm across) than the more advanced forms diagnosed 15 to 20 years ago.

"We are finding more and more breast cancers at an early, treatable stage," notes one radiologist, "probably because of greater cancer awareness, breast self-examination and thanks to mammography which detects the cancers before they are palpable [can be felt]." So conservative surgery to remove just the breast segment containing the tumor is becoming an increasingly accepted and safe option.

Several studies, including those done at Toronto's Princess Margaret Hospital and the large U.S. NSABP study – the National Surgical Adjuvant Breast and Bowel Project, involving 480 centers in North America – have confirmed that there is no survival advantage to any one type of breast surgery. Women who have breast-sparing lumpectomy live as long after diagnosis as those who have total breast removal. Whether women with breast cancer receive radical mastectomy, modified radical mastectomy or lumpectomy, survival figures are all the same.

"Broadly speaking," says one British cancer researcher, "we've moved from an era of mutilating supersurgery – the radical and supraradical mastectomies – to conservative surgery that requires postoperative radiotherapy and a willingness to accept a greater chance of local recurrence as the price of cosmetic acceptability." The current "state of the art" is breast-sparing surgery or lumpectomy followed by radiation for breast tumors under a certain size, with few exceptions (see Chapter 13). However, women who find the threat of local recurrence after lumpectomy unacceptable may prefer mastectomy, and it would also be advised for women who cannot have postoperative radiation because of illness or some other reason.

Adjuvant Therapy Is Now Usual after Surgery

Surgery alone does not guarantee a cure. Today's management focuses on breast cancer as a *systemic* disease, aiming to stop metastases with a "total body" attack. While some women never have a recurrence of cancer once the original breast tumor is removed, in many cases removal of the "primary" tumor is not enough. Microscopic malignant cells may have escaped (metastasized) and lodged elsewhere in the body, perhaps far from the original cancer, where they multiply and ultimately form another tumor that may not be detectable for years, even decades. Once these cancer cells have spread from the breast, no *local* remedy can stop them from growing into tumors. Therefore, systemic therapy is used after surgery to kill them, or to stop them from forming new tumor outposts elsewhere in the body. Most women with breast cancer now receive some form of postsurgical adjuvant therapy.

Adjuvant therapy can improve disease-free and overall survival in patients with positive (cancerous) underarm nodes. So today most lymph-node–positive women receive chemotherapy or hormone treatment. Until recently, node-negative women usually did not get systemic treatment, but study results in 1989 showed that adjuvant systemic therapy can improve disease-free survival even in node-negative patients. Therefore, many women with node-negative breast cancer now also receive postsurgical treatment. Postoperative drug treatment, formerly reserved for advanced metastatic disease, is now routinely offered to *all* node-positive women, and increasingly to node-negative women, particularly those thought to be at high risk of recurrence.

In deciding on the best treatment, physicians consider both the tumor characteristics and the state of the axillary nodes. *Radiation* to the operated breast is used to reduce local recurrences. *Chemotherapy* (with cancer-killing drugs) is used to destroy distant cancer cells elsewhere in the body. *Hormonal agents* such as tamoxifen are used to kill or retard the growth of hormone-dependent cancers. Sometimes ovary removal or ablation (destruction) is also tried. In general, chemotherapy is most often given to pre-menopausal women, while hormonal therapy is most likely to benefit post-menopausal women with hormone-receptor–bearing cancers, but there are no blanket rules.

Negative Lymph Nodes Are a Good Sign

One critical factor in predicting long-term survival is the presence of malignancy in the axillary (underarm) lymph nodes. Women have about 30 to 60 underarm nodes and surgeons generally remove 8 to 20 of the more accessible nodes, to be tested. If the lymph nodes test negative for cancer the chances are good for long-term, disease-free survival. Based on present statistics, 60 to 70 percent of women with breast cancer in North America are node-negative at diagnosis, while 30 to 40 percent have nodes showing signs of cancer. If the nodes contain cancerous cells, there's a high probability of spread to other parts of the body; if the lymph nodes test negative, there's about a 70 percent chance that no recurrence will occur (at least for many, many years). But 30 percent of node-negative women still relapse. "Paradoxically," notes one surgeon, "while the breast cancers found today are detected at an increasingly small size – under 2 to 3 cm [less than 1 inch] across – about 30 percent are *still* node-positive when discovered."

Even though women with small cancers and negative underarm nodes have the best outlook for both recurrence-free and overall survival, some women with ominous nodes at biopsy survive for many decades. Node-positive breast cancer has a relapse rate of 60 to 75 percent within ten years (compared to 30 percent for node-negative cases). The odds drop with more positive nodes. No positive lymph nodes indicates the most hopeful outlook; one to three is worse; four to ten is ominous and above ten the outlook is poor. The greater the number of positive lymph nodes, the lower the survival chances. (In future, staging systems with better markers may avoid the need for underarm node sampling.)

Controversy over Management of Node-negative Cases

Many oncologists believe that women with node-negative breast cancer should also receive adjuvant treatment. An alert from the U.S. National Cancer Institute recommends that they should "consider chemotherapy or hormone treatment." Other specialists disagree, saying that for node-negative patients the treatment decisions are far more complex. As one oncologist puts it, "We know that 70 percent of node-negative women who have early-stage tumors will do just fine with no systemic therapy, and only about 30 percent will relapse. So it is a philosophical question whether to put *all* node-negative women through not very pleasant drug therapy. Of course, for those who need it, it's a life-and-death decision." One approach is to give systemic therapy only to selected node-negative cases with a poor outlook. Scientists are trying to find specific tumor markers that show *which* node-negative cases need systemic treatment.

Staging and Prognosis

Once a cancer has been removed, its grade, stage and aggressivity are assessed before deciding on further treatment. Certain features signal a more aggressive or invasive cancer that calls for stronger treatment. For example, women with tumors rich in estrogen receptors (ERs) have more "breastlike" cancers and do slightly better (with longer disease-free survival) than those with no or few ERs. Tumors with cells not too actively dividing have a better prognosis than rapidly dividing ones.

Other features to be considered include:

- *age* – there is slightly more chance of local recurrence in younger women;
- *tumor size* – there is greater recurrence risk with larger cancers;
- *extent of the excision* – there is less risk of local recurrence with "wide margins," or plenty of normal breast tissue removed around the rim of the tumor. (There are still fewer recurrences after the more extensive "quadrantectomy" than after simple lumpectomy – see Chapter 13.)

Different Cancer Staging Systems

There are several systems for classifying, or "staging," the extent of breast cancer. The most common is the TNM system. In this system, T defines tumor size, N refers to the presence of cancer in the axillary nodes and M signifies the presence or absence of distant metastasis (spread).This system gives a rough estimate of the stage of the disease and is used as a guide to treatment. If there's suspicion that the cancer has spread, blood tests, X-rays, ultrasound and CT or bone scans can check for metastases in other organs. But the staging and tests cannot predict the outcome or prognosis for any *particular* woman, only her probable chances. Each case is unique.

The International TNM Classification Staging System for Breast Cancer can be summarized as follows:

- T0 = no primary tumor;
- Tis = cancer in situ;
- T1 = tumors up to 2 cm (0.8 inches) in size;
- T2 = tumors that measure 2 to 5 cm (0.8 to 2 inches) across;
- T3 = tumors over 5 cm in size;
- T4 = tumors of any size that extend to the chest wall or skin, including inflammatory breast cancer.

For the classification of the underarm nodes:

- N0 = no sign of cancer in the nodes;
- N1 = positive (cancerous) but mobile axillary nodes (not fixed);
- N2 = positive axillary nodes "fixed" to one another, or to other structures;
- N3 = positive axillary nodes with spread to internal mammary lymph node(s).

For the classification of metastases:

- M0 = no distant metastasis;
- M1 = distant metastasis (including spread to supraclavicular lymph nodes).

Staging a Cancer Tumor

Tumor

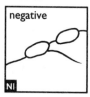

less than 2 cm

T1

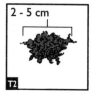

2 - 5 cm

T2

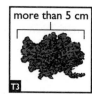

more than 5 cm

T3

extending to skin or chest wall

T4

Nodes

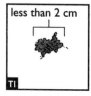

negative

N1

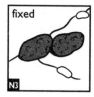

positive (mobile)

N2

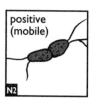

fixed

N3

fixed near collarbone

N4

Metastasis

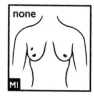

M1

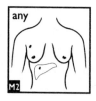

any

M2

Categorizing Breast Cancer by "Stages"

Stage 1: tumors under 2 cm in size, no positive nodes, no metastases;

stage 2: tumors 5 cm or less with some positive nodes, no metastases;

stage 3: tumors over 5 cm in size with positive, "fixed" nodes attached to skin or chest wall;

stage 4: metastatic cancer with distant spread (major sites are lung, bone, brain, liver).

Most breast cancers today are found at Stage 1 to 2, which means treatment can result in a good response. Stage 3 cancers sometimes respond to treatment, but not as often or as well as those treated at an earlier stage. Stage 4 cancers usually aren't curable, but they will often respond to treatment for a while and there is always a small chance they will temporarily remit or vanish.

Factors in Cancer Staging

- *Tumor size and pathological evaluation.*
- *Testing axillary lymph nodes.* Surgeons remove 8–20 armpit nodes for examination under a microscope. "Grossly positive" underarm nodes can often be felt and seen; axillary lymph nodes that are clearly swollen or can be felt, or are above the collarbone (*supraclavicular nodes*), generally signal metastatic cancer. "Microscopically positive" nodes show cancer only with a microscope examination.
- *Lung X-rays or a bone scan,* looking for signs of malignancy, possibly also a liver scan and, if there are strong suspicions of metastasis, a CAT (computerized axial tomography) scan.
- *Signs of advanced breast cancer* include:
  - swelling of the skin (edema) over the lump;
  - skin-dimpling, known as peau d'orange ("orange peel");
  - enlarged lymph nodes that can be felt;
  - angry, reddened skin around or over the breast lump; perhaps indicating inflammatory breast cancer.

Locally Advanced Breast Cancer

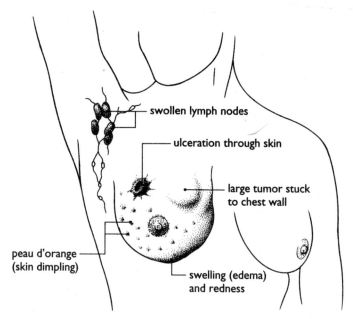

swollen lymph nodes

ulceration through skin

large tumor stuck to chest wall

peau d'orange (skin dimpling)

swelling (edema) and redness

Being "Informed" and Taking Part

Nowadays, decisions about the type of surgery to be done and the postoperative follow-up are often taken jointly by the woman and her caregivers. Although some women are comfortable knowing little about their cancer and its planned treatment, others wish to participate fully in their therapy. Many women want to know about the diagnosis, whether the cancer has spread, its stage, the chances of cure and the treatments available. Knowledge makes them feel more in control and "empowered." On the whole, women who receive clear, precise information about the disease and proposed treatments face the diagnosis better than those given little or no information.

"But some physicians are very patronizing," says one breast cancer activist, "and many women complain that they still get too little information from their doctors, or it's given in a hurried manner or makes them feel stupid."A diagnosis of breast cancer is liable to lay a woman open to all kinds of misinformation and scare-mongering. In the emotional aftermath of discovering they have cancer, women understandably feel vulnerable, helpless, scared and confused. People who get much of their health information from the media or word of mouth may be bewildered by the conflicting views expressed in books, magazines, TV and talk shows, or the personal anecdotes of friends, relatives and colleagues. A woman may feel relieved to hear about the benefits of a treatment offered, only to have her hopes shattered by a journalist who calls it "dangerously toxic," and perhaps castigates the medical establishment for using it, urging her "to fight back at all costs." It can be just as disconcerting to hear different opinions from various members of the caregiver team.

Treatment for breast cancer varies from place to place, depending on the knowledge, expertise and bias of the physicians. Since medical experts themselves disagree about the best treatment, it's no easy matter for women to find their way through the welter of conflicting opinions. They may find it baffling to learn that the treatment recommended for them differs from that given to a friend or relative. For example, a Vancouver woman who had a mastectomy and no postoperative treatment was surprised to learn that her cousin in Montreal had a lumpectomy followed by radiation and then chemotherapy, while a co-worker had a mastectomy and later had her ovaries removed. Of course, treatment *must* be tailored to the individual woman and the type and stage of her tumor, but not all women know this, or have it properly explained.

Foster Partnership with the Healthcare Team

At one time, women and their families were "silent members" of the healthcare team, if indeed they were considered partners at all. Today, people with cancer are encouraged to take an active role in their treatment, to develop good doctor-patient "partnerships," get to know the players and what each does. This can be challenging, as so many different specialists are involved. Try to find one member of the medical team whom you feel comfortable with, to serve as your guide and support – perhaps the oncologist, or one of the nurses, or your family doctor – and put crucial questions to him or her. You may feel you're being bombarded by alien information, but skilled professionals can usually simplify the facts and explain the alternatives at any stage of treatment. No matter how complex a problem may seem, the caregiver team can help women through the decision-making by giving the "big picture" and looking beyond the details to recovery.

Good Communication Helps Women Cope

People are more likely to feel satisfied with their care if they feel their concerns, grief and worry are taken seriously, and if caregivers acknowledge and empathize with their concerns. Good physician-patient communication is crucial for women dealing with breast cancer, to allow emotionally overwhelmed patients to learn about their disease, consider available treatments and participate in the decision-making. Several studies have addressed the way information – particularly bad news – is given to those with cancer, revealing huge gaps in patient recall and understanding. The news should never be given while a woman is still groggy from anesthesia, or be delivered inadvertently by a resident, pathologist or anyone other than the direct caregiver. A U.S. research group investigated the use of psychotherapeutic techniques by surgeons when informing women they had breast cancer, and found that certain techniques could help women adjust with less distress.

Physicians nowadays are urged to improve doctor-patient relationships, to become more "patient-friendly" and, above all, to improve their communication skills. The old authoritarian model of medical care is gradually giving way to a more "user-friendly" *biopsychosocial* model that encourages doctors to give people more information and consider the impact of illness and its treatment on their social, emotional and family life. "Empathy," explains one psychiatrist, "means listening not just to what the person says, but also to what's not said – bringing out the hidden agenda, the fears and worries." For example, patient hostility may mask anxiety; physicians need to understand and bring out the concerns that women wish to discuss. Given today's increasingly complex technology, health professionals prefer people to give "informed consent" to any tests or treatments undertaken. Surgeons and other doctors are advised to *verbalize* empathy, using simple statements such as "I know this news is very upsetting," and to give the woman "permission" to express emotions without feeling ashamed of being upset or tearful.

It's crucial for people to have sufficient time to absorb the news and react emotionally before the physician proceeds with more medical explanations. Communicating information is an *interactive* process between the woman and her caregivers.

Finding Reliable Information and the Right Doctor(s)

Many women are intimidated by doctors and hospitals. They're afraid to ask what awaits them or to discuss their concerns – unsure how to talk to physicians, reluctant to press for answers or for referral to another doctor. "The best idea," suggests a psychologist, "is to find one physician or caregiver whom you trust and feel comfortable with, and ask questions." Also find out as much as possible about the disease and up-to-date treatments from *reliable* sources, such as established local or federal cancer organizations, local breast screening or diagnostic centers or clinics, a trusted family physician, a breast specialist, the breast unit or oncology department of a large local hospital, or other staff who specialize in breast problems.

"Be consumer wise," suggests a member of the Canadian Breast Cancer Support Service, "but don't waste too much time doctor-shopping, hoping to hear what you'd like. Find a physician who suits your needs, someone who listens patiently and gives requested explanations. Ask questions about what worries you. Write them down so you don't forget and if not satisfied with the extent or manner of giving the answers, seek a second opinion." The surgeon selected should be a skilled operator, well trained in breast surgery. You may want to inquire whether he or she and the unit to which he or she is attached frequently treat women with breast cancer. Ask about the type of surgery planned and other treatments suggested. Do the clinic, hospital and its physicians favor a particular type of treatment, or is that determined case by case? In working with the oncologists after surgery, find ones who seem knowledgeable, willing to answer questions and share information with you in an open, understandable manner.

When going for medical visits, especially soon after diagnosis, have someone (friend, spouse, relative) accompany you to allay your anxiety, jog your memory about questions to ask and, above all, help remember what was said. Write down the answers to make sure you remember the information correctly – record any details about the type and size of breast cancer, test results and the stage of disease. The details of tests and treatments are often hard to memorize. Researchers have shown that, when someone sees a physician about an illness for the first time, approximately half the information is lost within 80 minutes, or by the time the person gets home.

Many women with breast cancer report *extreme* stress in the waiting periods – awaiting diagnosis and then awaiting radiation and other treatments. Some complain of a "com-

---

Questions to Ask about Breast Cancer

- What type and stage is my cancer?
- What treatments are recommended, and why?
- How does the treatment help, and how many women benefit?
- When, where and how often will treatments be given?
- What are the usual side effects? Will I feel bad?
- Are there any risks to the treatment?
- How long do the treatments take and go on for?
- What if I miss a treatment? Can I make it up?
- What will happen if I refuse this treatment?
- What problems should I report, and to whom?
- How can I contact the doctor(s) or medical team between visits?
- Can I take other medications or drink alcohol during treatment?

---

munication gap" or "void" after diagnosis, of being left frightened, with no one to talk to. Not surprisingly, the eventual treatment can come as a relief after all the waiting and uncertainty, allowing people to embark on the process of adjusting, coping and fighting the disease.

Counseling and Support Groups Can Help

Counselors, psychologists, dietitians and nurses attached to breast cancer, radiology or oncology units can be a help at these times, as can the family physician. Counselors experienced in the particular problems and challenges of cancer can be a particular help. Support and self-help groups can also be useful in coping with the disease, for those who wish to participate. Some women find that involvement with survivor networks or activist organizations is a constructive way to cope with the disease and feel more in control. Friends, relatives, lovers, spouses, children and companions of those with cancer also need emotional support in dealing with their fears. Nurses with special education and experience in counseling, social workers, psychologists and psychotherapists can give support. (See resource list at end of book.)

THIRTEEN

Surgical Options

Breast cancer operations today are far less drastic than
former methods – popularly dubbed the "cut, slash
and burn" approach – which removed the entire breast,
armpit contents and a large section of underlying muscle,
leaving the chest sunken and deformed and the arm badly
weakened. Nowadays, whenever possible, surgeons remove
just the tumor, leaving the rest of the breast intact.

Instead of breast removal or radical *mastectomy*, modern
breast cancer operations are mostly "breast-conserving
surgery" – removing just the cancerous lump and its surrounding margins, by a procedure called *lumpectomy*. Some
easily accessible axillary lymph nodes are also removed and
tested for cancer.

Changing Trends in Breast Surgery

The Halsted *radical mastectomy* was introduced about a
century ago by Dr. William Halsted, a U.S. surgeon who the-
orized that breast cancer spread "by direct extension along the
lymphatics, going from the breast directly to local then to
regional lymph nodes before affecting other parts of the body."

His operation left the breast badly deformed as it removed not only the tumor but the whole breast and nearby structures, including the pectoral muscles and many lymph nodes. While it reduced local recurrences, this drastic operation was rarely curative. Believing the operation didn't go far enough, surgeons removed yet another level of lymph nodes to try to improve cure rates. Having no luck, they added removal of the internal mammary lymph nodes (behind the breastbone), in what's known as an *extended radical mastectomy*. Later they also began removing the lymph nodes above the collarbone in a *supraradical mastectomy*. Although they were terribly disfiguring, these increasingly drastic surgical procedures gave no better survival figures. Clearly, surgery was no real cure for breast cancer.

With this realization, and the introduction of radiation during the 1940s, surgeons retreated from such destructive breast surgery. The *modified radical mastectomy* – removing far less tissue – produced equally good survival rates, with much less disability. Later, it became clear that removing just the tumor and saving the breast gave the same long-term survival as breast removal.

Today we know that for relatively small cancers, under about 4 cm (1 to 2 inches) across, survival rates are the same for lump-only removal as for mastectomy, provided lumpectomy is followed by radiation to the affected breast. In 1989 a U.S. National Institutes of Health (NIH) consensus conference proposed that less radical surgery become the standard procedure for breast cancer, saying that "Breast conservation is appropriate therapy for most women with Stage 1 and 2 breast cancer, providing survivals equivalent to total mastectomy while still preserving the breast." The NIH also recommended that the underarm lymph nodes be removed at the time of operation and that radiation to the operated breast routinely follow lumpectomy. Since more and more breast cancers are now found when relatively small, breast-conserving surgery is becoming more and more common.

The role of underarm node dissection has also changed. It is no longer done as a cure, since breast cancer does not necessarily spread through the lymph system. Instead, node removal is now used mainly to stage the cancer, to predict the outlook for survival and help physicians choose the best possible treatment. "If better methods come on board," notes one oncologist, "node removal for staging may be abandoned, particularly as it causes problems with numbness [due to damage or severing of underarm nerves] and lymphedema [fluid buildup], which can be very uncomfortable."

A Run-down of Today's Surgical Options
Partial mastectomy or *lumpectomy* removes just the tumor

Modified Radical Mastectomy

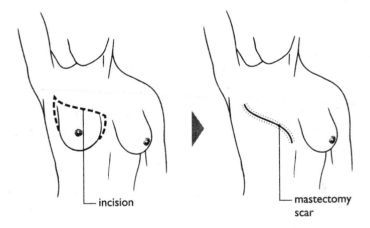

incision

mastectomy
scar

and some of the more accessible underarm nodes, leaving the rest of the breast intact, and is followed by postoperative radiation. Lumpectomy retains both a breast mound and the nipple and areola when possible. Surgeons excise extra breast tissue around the rim of the tumor to be sure all the cancer is out. The operation is done under general anesthesia, usually necessitating a hospital stay of four to five days to ensure that the scar is healing well and that there are no complications. Lumpectomy followed by radiation gives a woman the same chance of survival and local control of cancer as mastectomy, given a wide enough excision around the tumor.

Modified radical or *extended simple mastectomy* removes the whole breast and some armpit nodes. It is called "modified" because it removes less surrounding chest muscle than the Halsted operation. It is usually done under general anesthetic with a hospital stay of three to seven days. A "drain" or drainage tube is left in place to avoid fluid buildup. The scar is long and straight or diagonal across the chest wall.

Simple total mastectomy removes the breast but no muscles or axillary lymph nodes. It is done when there is no suspicion of cancer in the nodes – for example, as a preventive measure in women with a strong family history of breast cancer, who may decide to have both breasts removed to reduce the risk of developing the disease. A simple mastectomy may also be done for ductal carcinoma in situ, to prevent it from becoming invasive cancer later on.

Segmental mastectomy or *wide-excision mastectomy* removes the tumor and more normal breast tissue than a simple lumpectomy, but still leaves enough of a mound to give the breast a normal look.

Quadrantectomy removes one quarter of the breast and its skin.

A radical (Halsted) mastectomy is rarely done any more, but there are a few cases in which a toned-down version may be considered – for example, for a large tumor that has invaded the chest wall so that the only way to excise it completely is by removing part of the muscle as well as the breast and skin.

Axillary dissection usually accompanies breast cancer surgery. Surgeons generally remove the underarm nodes as a separate procedure after sewing up the first incision, for a neater look. Before closing the wound, the surgeon usually places a small drainage tube into the area where the lymph nodes were removed, to drain off any fluid that may collect. Studies show no survival benefit whatever the axillary node treatment – whether the underarm lymph nodes are removed, irradiated or left untouched – but node removal minimizes local recurrences in the armpit and provides the prognostic information needed for staging the cancer.

Deciding Jointly on the Needed Surgery

There are no absolute guidelines for deciding who should have lumpectomy versus mastectomy. Most surgeons nowadays do all they can to preserve a woman's breast, and choose the least extensive operation compatible with the extent of the disease. Since the choice of operation depends only partly on medical criteria, the decision about the "right surgery" is generally made in consultation with the woman and her family. The decision depends on the woman's preference and the surgeon's advice – which in turn depends on the size and type of tumor, its size in relation to the breast's size, its position in the breast (whether it is in the breast's ducts or lobes), and whether it is fixed or mobile, localized or invasive. Mastectomy may still be required for large tumors in a small breast, tumors that are advanced, immediately beneath or attached to the nipple, or in *multicentric* cases with several tumors in one breast. The tumor's location in the breast also counts. If it's in the middle

Choosing a Surgeon

Faced with cancer, many women are emotionally exhausted and leave the choice of surgeon to their family physician or the health professional who diagnosed the cancer. However, through lack of knowledge or bias, not all family physicians can or will refer women to the best available surgeon in their area. Some tend to refer them to the hospital to which they are attached or to a known colleague. "If you have a good relationship with your family doctor or have already discussed the problem with an oncologist," counsels one breast cancer expert, "request someone skilled in breast cancer surgery." Besides being skillful in operating techniques, the ideal surgeon is empathetic, listens attentively and explains things clearly. "But," notes one counselor, "this is a rare combination, and it's preferable to select a surgeon who specializes in breast operations, rather than one with a warm bedside manner." Information about local surgeons can be obtained from agencies such as the Reach to Recovery program of the Canadian Cancer Society, or from local breast screening clinics, health departments, support and advocacy groups for breast cancer or nurses at the local cancer clinic or hospital.

of the breast, the nipple may have to be removed, giving a poor cosmetic result; again, mastectomy may be preferable. But reconstructive breast surgery, done at the same time as mastectomy or later, can restore both a breast and a nipple for women who desire it.

In general, lumpectomy is suggested for women with small breast cancers less than 4 cm (1 to 2 inches) across, with no evidence of spread to the skin, bone, lungs or other sites. For large tumors, the size of the breast must be carefully considered. Tumors larger than 5 cm (2 inches) are generally removed by modified radical mastectomy.

Proof That Lumpectomy Really Works

"While it's nice to be able to tell women with breast cancer they can have a lumpectomy and don't need the whole breast removed," notes one University of Toronto surgeon, "I like to tell them *why* it's no longer considered necessary to take off the breast. The proof that lumpectomy and mastectomy give equal survival chances comes mainly from a huge U.S. trial done in the mid-1970s – the National Surgical Adjuvant Breast and Bowel Project or NSABP '06' study – which conclusively showed that the chances of cure, or ten-year survival (which is our best guess at cure), were the same whether the whole breast or just the cancerous lump was removed."

This NSABP study took 2,000 women with breast cancer and assigned them randomly to one of three treatment groups:

- *mastectomy* – removal of the whole breast and some underarm lymph nodes;
- *lumpectomy* – "lump only" removal and removal of some underarm nodes;
- *lumpectomy plus radiation* to the operated breast afterwards.

Overall survival was absolutely equivalent in all three groups.

Lumpectomy

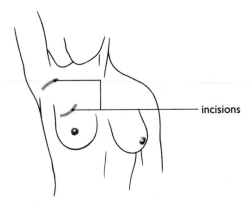

incisions

But women who received no radiation after lumpectomy had a high local cancer recurrence rate on the operated side, even though there was no diminution in overall survival. "This means," explains the surgeon, "that if radiation is not given after lumpectomy there's an unacceptably high rate of local recurrence – about 25 to 40 percent – which is reduced to 8 to 10 percent given a postsurgical course of radiotherapy to the operated side." Radiation is now usually advised after lumpectomy.

Pros and Cons of Lumpectomy

The advantages of lumpectomy are less extensive surgery, fewer postsurgical after-effects, keeping the breast, avoiding the need for a prosthesis (artificial breast form) and less psychological trauma – less erosion of self-image, sense of femininity and self-esteem. In addition, once word gets around that breast cancer doesn't necessarily mean losing a breast, women may be more inclined to seek medical advice promptly if they discover a lump, rather than delaying as so often happens – sometimes with tragic results.

The disadvantages of lumpectomy are the need for post-surgical radiation, the need for more careful and thorough checkups, and possibly greater worry about local recurrence. Women who have lumpectomies must consider the somewhat greater chances of recurrence and their ability to cope with daily radiation for four weeks, although radiation sessions take only 10 to 15 minutes a day. (See Chapter 14 for more on radiotherapy.)

Follow-up after Lumpectomy

Curiously, although lumpectomy was thought to make women "feel better," studies show that the psychological advantages of lumpectomy versus mastectomy are less striking than expected. That's largely because, although the breast is preserved, it's at the cost of greater fears of recurrence.

The woman must have her affected breast regularly and carefully checked to detect cancer recurrence on that side. She should get to know the normal feel of her treated breast. After the radiation, there can be areas of scarring – hardness or lumpiness – and these must be monitored. The best way for a woman to continue keeping tabs on her breasts is by monthly breast self-examination and by having a clinical examination every six months by a skilled healthcare professional. She should also have a mammogram six months after the radiation treatment ends, followed by mammograms of both breasts once a year or so, as advised by her physician.

Mastectomy Is Still Sometimes Necessary

Not all women with breast cancer can be offered lumpectomy. The cosmetic results can be displeasing, even disastrous, if lumpectomy is tried in inappropriate cases. If the tumor is large and the breast small, it may remove so much tissue that the breast is distorted and the cosmetic result is a bitter blow. In such cases mastectomy is preferable.

Pros and Cons of Mastectomy

The advantages of mastectomy are no need for postoperative radiation, slightly lower chances of cancer recurring in the operated breast and, for some women, a feeling of having done "the most possible" toward a cure.

The disadvantages of mastectomy are losing a breast, readjustment of body-image – sometimes long and hard – embarrassment at letting others see the disfigurement, the constant anatomical reminder of having a potentially lethal disease and reduced choices of clothing or "cleavage-showing" garments. Even after a mastectomy, given a good prosthesis or skillful breast reconstruction, women can dress in low necklines or swimsuits to look just as they did before breast removal. With the aid of artistry and carefully chosen garments no one need know that they lack a breast.

A mastectomy may seem the best solution for a woman whose breasts are always lumpy and who is "never going to trust that breast." Some women choose mastectomy because, after evaluating the options, they believe it's the only way they'll feel able to "relax." Others don't want the radiation therapy required after lumpectomy. Studies show that the anxiety levels of women after breast surgery depend largely on the type of information they are given and the way it is given – in a curt and hurried or friendly, leisurely manner. Surveys suggest that women may feel greater anxiety after lumpectomy than after mastectomy, depending on individual character and life situations. Other studies show that preserving the breast greatly enhances a woman's quality of life and self-image. In one study, a year after breast surgery, women had similar levels of distress regardless of whether they had their

Timing Surgery in Tune with the Body's Cycle

Since several recent studies have shown that breast cancer surgery at different points in the cycle can give varying outcomes, pre-menopausal women are often advised to have their operation in the second half of the menstrual cycle. Women operated on during days 3 to 12 of the menstrual cycle (day one being the first day of the period) had on average a 54 percent chance of surviving for ten years, compared to 84 percent if surgery was performed later in the cycle. The difference was most marked among women with positive underarm nodes, for whom surgery in the second half of the cycle more than doubled the ten-year survival rate. One explanation could be hormonal; during the early part of the cycle estrogen levels are high and progesterone levels are low. Perhaps cancer cells released into the body during surgery survive better in a particular hormonal environment. However, other studies have failed to show the same effect.

breast removed or saved. In other words, cancer causes stress, no matter what type of surgery is done.

Management of Advanced Breast Cancer

Surgery is not always the first treatment for cancers that are advanced – for example, very large tumors or very enlarged lymph nodes, or inflammatory cancer. In such situations, chemotherapy and radiation may be given first to reduce the size of the tumor, and mastectomy may follow. When there is evidence of metastatic cancer beyond the breast, the initial treatment may include hormones, chemotherapy and radiation, rather than surgery. In this situation the cancer beyond the breast is the greater threat and requires urgent treatment.

How Are Cancers in Situ Treated?

Paradoxically, breast-sparing surgery may *not* be the best choice for some non-invasive, early breast cancers. Early *carcinomas in situ* – "in place," not yet invading adjacent tissues – are regarded more as markers for future cancer than as true cancers. However, there is a high likelihood that cancer in situ will become invasive, and this poses a treatment dilemma: should physicians simply follow the woman closely and hope to detect signs of invasiveness?

Curiously, although less radical surgery is now the norm for most small breast cancers, there's considerable debate about the right treatment for cancers in situ. Many specialists suggest partial mastectomy or lumpectomy (with or without radiation) as the best management, excising just the calcified area but not the underarm nodes. Others favour total mastectomy as a preventive measure, rather than "waiting for the cancer to grow." Those with in situ cancers who opt for breast-sparing surgery may have to live with a certain level of uncertainty, while those who choose mastectomy can have breast reconstruction.

After the Operation

Apart from the surgical changes to a woman's breast, there can be some annoying after-effects following breast cancer operations. Breast tissue usually heals fast and well, but there may be some bruising and swelling immediately after the operation.

Postoperative pain is common at first, along the incision and under the arm, and is controlled with pain medication such as acetaminophen or ASA. Later, there may be some tightness or discomfort over the chest area – usually mild but occasionally bothersome.

The incision usually heals within a few weeks, but healing may take longer in women who have had radiation before surgery. Chemotherapy can also delay healing. Care of the incision is explained in hospital, and women can usually shower within a week.

Wound infections are infrequent. Danger signs include a foul smell, an increasingly red and tender scar or a fever – symptoms to report and treat promptly, usually with antibiotics.

Drainage tubes are removed before the woman leaves hospital or a few days later, depending on the amount of fluid and the length of the hospital stay. Sometimes fluid builds up after the drain tubes come out, and can be drained with a syringe in the surgeon's office. Or it can come back later and be annoyingly persistent. (See Chapter 15 for advice about this.)

Stitches (sutures) may dissolve on their own, but some types or staples need to be removed, usually a week to ten days after surgery. Ask the surgeon what sort of sutures will be used.

Numbness in the back of the underarm or in the chest wall can occur due to underarm nerves being cut or stretched during the operation. Sensation generally returns in a few months to a year, depending on the extent of surgery, but if certain underarm nerves have been cut numbness may persist.

Instability and "winging" of the shoulder blades used to be a problem when the nerve supply to muscles in the base of the armpit was damaged in radical breast surgery. This is now rare.

Weakness or stiffening of the shoulder and arm is common, and arm movements may be difficult for a while. The muscles must be rebuilt by special arm exercises taught by a physiotherapist. Radical mastectomy was notorious for causing a stiff arm because muscles were removed, but now that this operation is rarely done severe postoperative arm problems have largely disappeared. Nevertheless, women still need special exercises – learned from a physiotherapist – to restore full arm and shoulder flexibility (see Chapter 15 for details).

FOURTEEN

Postsurgical Therapy

After surgery to remove a breast tumor, women are generally referred to oncologists for further advice and treatment, perhaps at a specialized cancer center or clinic. The *radiation oncologist* administers radiotherapy (radiation therapy) and the *medical oncologist* usually plans and supervises drug and hormone therapy. The choice of postoperative adjuvant treatment is based on the size, type, stage and invasiveness of the cancer, and the woman's age. The treatment usually starts a few weeks after surgery, once the wound has healed. These days, adjuvant therapy is routinely offered to *all* node-positive women and increasingly to certain node-negative cases. New recommendations are constantly being developed to keep pace with the results of trials, and as we gain new insights into the biology of cancer.

Postoperative Breast Cancer Treatments
Adjuvant treatments include:

- *radiation* – used after lumpectomy to reduce chances of local recurrence and destroy local metastases;

- *hormonal treatment* with anti-estrogens or other agents;
- *ovary removal or ablation* (destruction) to slow or halt hormone-dependent tumor growth;
- *chemotherapy* with various cytotoxic (cell-killing) drugs to destroy lingering cancer cells anywhere in the body.

Who Should Get What Postoperative Treatment?

Experts still argue the crucial questions in breast cancer: who should get what postsurgical treatment, which kind and for how long? Most physicians agree on the need for radiation after lumpectomy, and chemotherapy is a frequent choice for pre-menopausal women, while hormonal therapy often seems most effective for older women, especially those with hormone-receptor–bearing tumors. But there are no hard and fast rules; therapy is individually tailored to the woman and her tumor. In general:

- *pre-menopausal, node-positive women* get chemotherapy with several drugs;
- *post-menopausal, node-positive women* whose tumors possess hormone receptors receive the anti-estrogen tamoxifen, or other anti-hormone agents such as goserelin acetate;
- *node-negative cases* receive varied therapy. Many oncologists now recommend adjuvant treatment for node-negative cases, especially those with "bad" tumor features and a poor outlook, with either hormone therapy or chemotherapy.

As already noted, oncologists still argue about the best treatment for node-negative women. Approximately seven out of ten women with no cancer in their underarm nodes will be cured by breast-saving surgery plus radiation alone. But in the other three out of ten cases, the cancer will recur even though the lymph nodes appear to be cancer-free. That's why it's critical to look at other factors to identify the women at greatest risk of relapse. For instance, node-negative women with small tumors low in estrogen receptors (ERs) – who therefore respond poorly to hormone therapy – may not be considered at high enough risk to merit the unpleasant effects of chemotherapy.

A Sample Treatment Plan:

- chemotherapy for all node-positive pre-menopausal cases;
- tamoxifen for two to five (or more) years for node-positive, post-menopausal women whose cancers are estrogen-receptor–positive (ER-positive) or progesterone-receptor-positive (PgR-positive);
- ovary removal or ablation (destruction) for node-positive, pre-menopausal, ER- or PgR-positive women unwilling or unable to have other therapy (or who prefer ovarian surgery);
- chemotherapy for node-negative, pre- and post-menopausal women with ER-negative tumors (in selected cases);
- tamoxifen for node-negative, post-childbearing women with ER-bearing tumors and no "bad" prognostic features;
- the LHRH hormone-inhibitor goserelin acetate (Zoladex) for some high-risk node-negative cases.

Radiation Therapy (Radiotherapy)

Radiation therapy uses high-energy X-rays from special machines to kill cancer cells and shrink tumors. Radiotherapy is usually given for 21 to 25 days over a period of three to five weeks. Each session lasts a few minutes, once an initial planning session has determined the site and dose of radiation. The exact area to be irradiated is marked with a tattoo pen. An extra "boost" is often given to the scar area. The X-rays only penetrate the small targeted area where the cancer is located.

Breast Cancer Treatment Plan Based on 1995 St. Gallen Consensus Conference

	NODE-NEGATIVE CASES			NODE-POSITIVE CASES	
	Minimal Risk (Grade 1 tumors, under 1 cm in size)	**Low Risk** 1–2 cm in size; (Grades 1–2, ER +ve)	**High Risk** >1 cm, ER –ve, or >2 cm, ER +ve, or Grade 3 (high)	**Hormone-Receptor Negative**	**Hormone-Receptor Positive**
Pre-menopausal	tamoxifen or nil? (unclear)	tamoxifen, (ovary removal? or chemo?) possibly LHRH (Zoladex)?	receptor +ve: chemo; (? also tamoxifen, or ovary removal, or LHRH?) receptor –ve: chemo	chemo with AC or CMF	chemo with AC or CMF; (+/– ovary removal, tamoxifen? LHRH?)
Post-menopausal	tamoxifen or nil? (unclear)	tamoxifen	receptor +ve: tamoxifen; (+/– chemo?) receptor –ve: chemo; (+/– tamoxifen)	chemo with AC or CMF (possibly also tamoxifen? sequentially?)	tamoxifen (possibly also chemo? sequentially?)
Elderly	?nothing	tamoxifen	tamoxifen; (or possibly chemo if ER –ve)	tamoxifen or chemo	tamoxifen

?: not standard treatment, but for research to decide; unclear
LHRH: Zoladex (goserelin acetate)
ER +ve: estrogen-receptor positive

chemo: chemotherapy
AC: Adriamycin (doxorubicin) + cyclophosphamide
CMF: cyclophosphamide + methotrexate + 5-fluorouracil

receptor –ve: hormone-receptor negative
receptor + ve: hormone-receptor positive
ER –ve: estrogen-receptor negative

They do not stay in the body or travel around it, do not make the person radioactive, and there is no danger in kissing, cuddling or lovemaking. Radiotherapy does not cause infertility (unless the ovaries are irradiated as part of treatment), and it doesn't make the hair fall out (unless the head is irradiated). The radiation does not hurt, and is much like having a normal X-ray except that it lasts a bit longer; the woman must lie or sit still during it. Fortunately, in contrast to fast-dividing cancer cells that shrivel up from the effects of radiation, normal cells repair themselves quickly and completely after any radiation damage. Since the radiation is given in a series of small treatments, normal cells recover between treatments while the cancer cells die off.

Although radiation undoubtedly lessens the chances of recurrence, it hasn't been shown to extend overall survival, and doctors debate the necessity of giving it to *all* women who have lumpectomies. Oncologists would prefer to have a way to pick out women with particularly aggressive tumors at high risk of recurrence and give them the radiotherapy, saving the others from it. A large trial is now under way to look into this possibility. "We wonder," speculates one radiation oncologist, "whether there is a subgroup of people who don't really need radiotherapy after lumpectomy, for instance older women with very small cancers, who could be managed as effectively with a wide local excision and tamoxifen to curb recurrences." But this remains an experimental approach.

Radiotherapy may also be suggested for women who have had modified radical mastectomies for large tumors, and for inflammatory cancers that penetrate the skin. It may also be given for locally advanced, or diffuse, inoperable breast cancers, and to relieve symptoms of metastatic spread in the bones or other sites. Radiation for a recurrent tumor cannot later be repeated in the same spot (because normal tissues are

Radiation Therapy

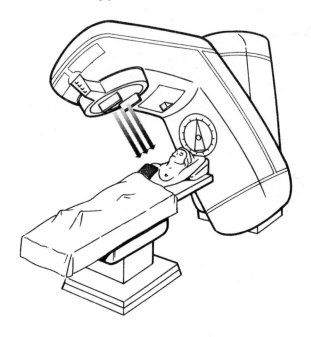

already sensitized and could be damaged), but if a new cancer develops elsewhere it can be considered for radiotherapy. Lymph node areas aren't usually irradiated.

Tips for Coping with Radiotherapy

"Forewarned is forearmed," so most women cope best with radiation therapy if they know exactly what to expect. Ask the caregivers when the treatment will begin, where it will take place, how long it will continue, what it entails and what side effects may occur. For the skin reddening or irritation, keep the area dry, don't wash off the ink marks and avoid use of greasy ointments. Discuss skin care with your oncologist. Most women report very little disturbance in their usual routine,

---

Side Effects of Radiation:

- slight to moderate skin redness (like a sunburn) and possible darkening (pigmentation) – especially in the fair-skinned – which sometimes lingers after radiotherapy ends;
- fatigue, especially toward the end of the course, perhaps partly due to the effort of traveling to and from the therapy so often. It's a good idea to have a short rest after each treatment;
- fibrosis (scarring) and hardening of the breast and underlying tissue, sometimes permanent;
- edema or fluid collection in the arm area, due to node removal, possibly worsened by irradiation;
- occasional breast tenderness, requiring a softer bra (which can persist for a while after therapy ends);
- sometimes short-lived coughing or shortness of breath because of lung scarring due to radiation scatter;
- slight chance of damage to the heart and marginally elevated cardiac risks, in those who have *left-sided* breast irradiation (rare).

---

other than fatigue. However, the fatigue can make housework and food preparation burdensome, so it's a good idea to have on hand a variety of convenience foods for preparing simple but nutritious meals – a sandwich, hearty soup and toast, or a bowl of cereal with milk and fruit may be ample. Because radiation involves the chest area, people may develop a temporary sore throat, cough or lung irritation. Eating soft, moist foods is helpful, such as poached eggs, creamed fish, chicken stew, fruit yogurt or blended foods. Very hot or spicy foods such as curry, tea or soup can make a sore throat worse.

Chemotherapy: "Present Pain for Future Gain"

Chemotherapy uses various cytotoxic (cell-killing) agents in an attempt to eradicate any remaining cancer cells and those that have spread from the breast. "It is best," says one breast surgeon, "to tell women well ahead about possible side effects of chemotherapy – remove the mystery and take out the bogeymen – before starting treatment, as people have heard awful stories and are very frightened of it. But chemotherapy can substantially improve survival and even cure the cancer in some cases." Urging women to look ahead and think of the drugs killing the cancer cells, she calls it "present pain for future gain."

Common side effects include nausea, dry mouth, diarrhea, gritty eyes, blurred vision, heartburn (gastric reflux), bladder irritation, vomiting, hair loss, insomnia, sexual disturbances, fatigue, a lowered white-blood-cell count, heart irregularities and, understandably, anxiety. Side effects vary considerably from person to person with the chemotherapy regime. *Drug-induced amenorrhea* (cessation of periods and reduced estrogen release) occurs in about half the women under age 40 (and more over-40s) undergoing chemotherapy, and may result in permanent infertility. Once the "chemo" ends, most side effects gradually vanish, but it can take months to get over the fatigue and feel "back to normal" again.

The potent chemotherapy drugs temporarily affect healthy tissue, which explains some of their side effects. The drugs "poison" rapidly dividing cancer cells and also transiently affect other fast-dividing cells in the body, such as the hair follicles, blood-producing cells and the lining of the stomach and bladder. That's why the hair may fall out, the white-blood-cell count may drop and people experience nausea or bladder irritation. But while the cytotoxic drugs *kill* cancer cells, their effect on normal cells is usually temporary. Once the "chemo" is over, the body recuperates and regains its normal function: the hair grows back, the nausea vanishes and the blood normalizes.

Different chemotherapy drugs work in different ways, and people react differently to them. The type of chemotherapy most commonly used for breast cancer is CMF – a mixture of three drugs, *cyclophosphamide methotrexate* and *5-fluorouracil* (5-FU). Other drugs include *doxorubicin* (Adriamycin) and *epirubicin*. Common drug combinations used include:

- AC – Adriamycin (doxorubicin) and cyclophosphamide;
- CAF (or FAC) – cyclophosphamide, Adriamycin and 5-fluorouracil;
- CEF – cyclophosphamide, epirubicin and 5-FU.

Postoperative chemotherapy is usually given for three to six months, by mouth or injection, with intervals of three to four weeks between doses to reduce the toxicity. Since the therapy tends to lower levels of white blood cells (needed to fight infection), a blood test is taken before each bout of "chemo" to ensure that the blood chemistry has recuperated and can withstand the drugs. If the white-cell count is too low, the next dose is delayed until the blood count climbs back to a safe level. The cardiotoxicity or possible effects on the heart are also closely monitored.

The side effects of "chemo" are often debilitating and women usually have to rest for a few hours, or even a day, after each chemotherapy session. But many manage to go on working and even exercising through their chemotherapy courses. Most side effects are predictable, but a few are not. For example, some chemotherapy drugs always cause hair loss while others rarely affect the hair. In the last few years several drugs have been developed that produce fewer side effects; and other drugs, given alongside the chemotherapy drugs, can minimize side effects.

Chemotherapy gives an overall 25 to 28 percent reduction in the yearly recurrence rate and a 16 to 20 percent reduction in the annual death rate from breast cancer.

Although chemotherapy is usually given after surgery, in a few centers it is sometimes given, on an experimental basis, before surgery, to shrink the tumor. Trials are under way to compare pre- and postoperative chemotherapy. Combined chemotherapy and hormonal therapy, with chemotherapy and hormones used one after the other or together, may still further improve survival rates, and this possibility is also being tested.

Tips for Coping with Chemotherapy

If women understand why they need chemotherapy and what to expect, it is easier for them to accept the side effects. Once chemotherapy ends, the body recovers and the unpleasant effects will ultimately vanish. But it can take weeks, even months, to get back to normal so women who still feel weak, tired and "down" after therapy ends shouldn't despair – the effects *will* gradually fade.

During chemotherapy, nausea, a sore mouth, taste changes and mild diarrhea are common. Nausea is best controlled by specific medications and certain foods; many centers give an antinauseant along with the chemotherapy, and most units have specialized dietitians on tap to give advice. Don't hesitate to ask for help from the support staff. If the smell of cooking worsens the nausea, avoid being in the kitchen if possible, and stock up on ready-made items or homemade frozen dinners that can be easily reheated. Foods low in fiber can help to offset stomach upsets and diarrhea. Starchy foods, plain white rather than very grainy breads and cereals, and crackers and dry cereals nibbled often can help minimize nausea. Fluids such as flat ginger ale, weak tea, diluted fruit juice or plain ice water are generally better tolerated than milk, shakes, coffee or very sweet juices. Keeping a thermos or giant cup close by can help remind a woman to drink plenty during chemotherapy.

Mild diarrhea and gas can be minimized by limiting intake of fiber-rich foods and avoiding bowel stimulants such as alcohol and caffeine. Excess gas can be partially controlled by eating less gas-forming food such as legumes, cabbage, Brussels sprouts, melons, apples and grapes. Most breast treatment clinics or oncology units can provide information about the best diet and management of side effects. Individual counseling and support groups can be a great help for the many who feel in need of help.

Hormonal Therapy

Hormone treatment works by lowering hormone levels or blocking their impact and by slowing the growth of hormone-sensitive cancers or killing them. Through the years, many hormonal (endocrine) strategies have been tried, including removal of the ovaries, adrenals and/or pituitary glands, as well as the administration of anti-hormonal agents such as anti-estrogens, LHRH (luteinizing hormone-releasing factor) blockers (such as goserelin acetate) and anti-progestins (like RU-486). The therapy selected depends on whether the tumor has *estrogen receptors* (ER), *progesterone receptors* (PgR) or both. The discovery of these hormone-sensitive receptors in breast tumor cells has improved the fine-tuning and effectiveness of treatment.

Ovarian Destruction

The traditional use of ovarian ablation (removal or suppression) to reduce the tumor-promoting influence of estrogens is once more gaining favor in some centers for pre-menopausal breast cancers. In some pre-menopausal women, ovarian ablation – by surgery or radiation – can increase disease-free and overall survival. (By contrast, adrenal and pituitary removal are rarely used any more for breast cancer treatment.)

Stopping the secretion of estrogens from the ovaries by removing them surgically or destroying them with radiation can increase survival rates by 10 to 15 percent at 15-year follow-up, but physicians hesitate to destroy or remove the ovaries of young women because of long-term side effects – premature menopause, infertility and increased risk of heart disease and osteoporosis. "Yet," notes one oncologist, "when we give chemotherapy it anyway leads to cessation of periods and ovulation in almost half the young women who take it, which amounts almost to the same thing – although it's more gradual."

Tamoxifen Remains the Treatment Mainstay

Tamoxifen is one of today's most commonly used treatments for breast cancer. It is an anti-estrogen with few side effects. But while it is well tolerated by most women, its adverse effects must be considered and the pros and cons carefully discussed before treatment is undertaken.

Tamoxifen has been shown to reduce the chance of cancer in the opposite breast by 40 percent. A daily 20 mg tablet, taken for two to five years, gives a 20 percent drop in the risk of dying from breast cancer. The protective effect apparently persists for at least ten years. It can benefit all women but its impact seems to be most effective in those whose tumors have many hormone receptors, in both pre- and post-menopausal cases.

In general, the higher the estrogen-receptor level, the more responsive the cancer will be to tamoxifen. If the pathologist reports few or no ERs in a tumor, it's not likely to respond. "But," warns one oncologist, "reports stating an absence of ERs may be inaccurate and the tumor may in fact have a few receptors and respond to tamoxifen to some extent." Although its exact mechanism isn't clear, tamoxifen seems to act both as a weak estrogenic female hormone and as an anti-estrogen that binds to part of the tumor's estrogen-receptor sites, blocking the cancer-promoting effects of the body's own estrogen. It may also directly halt tumor expansion by stimulating the release of a cancer-growth inhibitor.

Many studies have convincingly shown that tamoxifen can improve disease-free and overall survival in post-menopausal women with ER-bearing tumors. An analysis of world data done at Britain's Oxford University – known as the "Oxford Overview" – confirmed that tamoxifen can prolong survival. Although it seems to be most beneficial in post-menopausal women, studies are also investigating its use in younger women (perhaps in addition to chemotherapy).

Tamoxifen is increasingly tried for node-negative as well as for node-positive cases. "Since even among the node-negative cases 30 percent have recurrences in ten years," explains one oncologist, "any survival benefits are worth a try. We think tamoxifen may be as useful as chemotherapy in certain node-negative cases with aggressive tumors." Tamoxifen is also being tried as a cancer-preventive in high-risk women (see Chapter 20).

The optimal duration of tamoxifen treatment and the length of time for which it can safely be taken are much-debated questions. Most oncologists recommend that women who feel comfortable with the drug take it for two years, sometimes five to ten years, or indefinitely, but resistance to the drug can develop after a year or two.

The Balance Sheet on Tamoxifen Use

- It increases *disease-free survival* in pre- and post-menopausal women – most significantly in node-positive, post-menopausal women with hormone receptors in their cancers.

Possible Side Effects of Tamoxifen

Although many women tolerate tamoxifen well and experience no side effects, others have noticeable problems, such as:

- hot flashes – often transient;
- vaginal discharge (very common);
- continuation or return of menstruation;
- nausea or vomiting, loss of appetite – rare and usually temporary;
- weight gain;
- endometrial (uterine lining) hyperplasia (thickening) that can lead to cancer. Women with an intact uterus who take tamoxifen have a two to three times higher than average risk of endometrial cancer, so the risks and benefits must be carefully weighed if women stay on tamoxifen for several years. (There are three cases of endometrial cancer per thousand women who take tamoxifen for five or more years);

In general the benefits greatly outweigh the risks.

- *It can reduce the risk of recurrence in the affected breast and of tumor development* in the other breast by 40 percent.
- *Its short-term side effects* are generally mild and well tolerated, although it triggers or worsens hot flashes.
- *It seems to protect against heart disease*, by lowering "bad" (LDL) blood cholesterol and raising "good" (HDL) cholesterol, and may protect against the bone loss that causes osteoporotic fractures. The head of one major cancer center notes that "taking tamoxifen may actually have effects similar to HRT – hormone replacement therapy – in protecting women against cardiovascular disease and postmenopausal bone loss."
- *The main long-term side effect* is the increased risk of endometrial cancer in those taking it for a few years.

The Search for a "Better Tamoxifen"

New anti-estrogens that act like tamoxifen are being tested to see if they have fewer side effects and greater effectiveness. For example, droloxifene, toremifene and trioxifene have some anti-cancer effects.

What's on the Horizon in Anti-Cancer Strategies:

- *better definition of groups that can most benefit* from specific treatments or those who don't need any at all;
- *new steroidal anti-estrogens* similar to tamoxifen but with fewer risks and side effects, now in clinical trials;
- *innovative tests* to help identify patients who might benefit most from hormone or chemotherapy, for instance DNA *flow cytometry* and *neu-oncogene* (cancer-gene) measurements (still experimental);
- *a synthetic hormone (anti-estrogen), somatostatin,* that can halt tumor growth;
- *LHRH agonists* like *buserelin, leuprolide* or *goserelin acetate,* which may maintain remission in pre-menopausal women by shutting down their ovaries;
- *new methods of ovary oblation* (destruction) instead of removal;
- *new chemotherapy drugs, in special high-dose regimens;* new combinations and drug schedules;
- *delaying surgery until after the breast tumor has been shrunk* with powerful doses of chemotherapy and radiation;
- *an agent from Pacific yew bark* – Taxol, or a synthetic relative of Taxol, docetaxel (taxotere) – containing diacetyl baccitin as the active ingredient, which can retard tumor growth, used alongside other drugs. Side effects include some hair loss, muscular aches and changes in blood counts;
- *topical capsaicin,* the active ingredient in hot peppers, which

can help reduce post-mastectomy pain;

- *autologous bone-marrow or stem-cell transplants* (taken from the woman's own body), with promising results in advanced cases. The body is given extremely high doses of chemotherapy, after "harvesting" of some bone marrow or stem (blood-forming) cells. Once the potent drugs have obliterated all cancer cells, the harvested blood-forming cells are reinfused into the bloodstream to regenerate the blood-forming system; but because of the vast doses of chemotherapy given, the woman's body remains very vulnerable to infection for several weeks – a key danger of the procedure, which has a considerable mortality rate;
- *weight control and dietary strategies* – especially to prevent recurrences.

Finding Accurate Information to Aid Recovery

Women undergoing treatment for breast cancer need specific information and reassurance. For instance, they need to know that radiation is not permanently harmful, although a few side effects such as skin sensitivity can linger on. Those having chemotherapy must be prepared for the hair loss, nausea and other effects, and know how to combat them – buy a wig, take antinauseants – and know that the side effects are temporary and that the hair will grow back, and the body eventually recover, although it takes time.

Having precise information can help to allay the natural anxiety and uncertainties involved in treatment. Women usually have many questions to ask and worries to inquire about, and often don't know where to turn. However, most oncology and breast cancer units have counselors, specialized nurses, psychologists and others who can answer questions and give friendly advice. Try to find them!

Studies show that women whose caregivers fully discuss treatment with them are less anxious and suffer less depression than women not offered the chance of discussion, irrespective of the operation they had. Having explored all the available treatment options, and found the pros and cons of each, most women move into a "get-on-with-it" stage, ready to accept and cope with treatment and, although maybe not happy about the situation, no longer in shock.

The local chapters of cancer societies are good places to obtain information, advice and help. Most provide booklets, seminars and stress management training and can guide people to self-help groups. Specialized counseling is often an enormous help during the stressful period of cancer therapy. Cancer information hotlines with 1-800 numbers can be called for advice, free of charge. Survivor organizations are also good places to seek information and support.

In coping with the treatments, support from friends, family, colleagues and empathetic health professionals can help. Many family members feel afraid they won't know how to talk or relate to people with cancer, but once the "ice is broken" it should not be too difficult to just "be there" for the person. Joining self-help or other support groups can help in facing the implications of having cancer. "Above all," advises one specialist, "women should select caregivers they trust and can share worries with, being prepared to seek further expert opinions if need be." (See resource list at end of book.)

FIFTEEN

Recovery and Follow-up

In the immediate aftermath of discovering they have breast cancer and dealing with the surgery and other treatments, people are generally in a numb state of shock. During the immediate postoperative treatment period, while coping with the hassle, unknowns and side effects of therapy – which can all be very frightening – there's little time to dwell on the deeper emotional and existential aspects of cancer. Usually, women only begin to realize the full implications once therapy ends and recovery is under way.

To some extent, dealing with the practicalities of treatment, after the strain of awaiting diagnosis, can dissipate the shock and helplessness and bring a sense of relief in "doing something" – discussing options with the medical team, deciding on the details of therapy, coping with the often under-explained and unexpected side effects. The treatments for breast cancer may go on for months, with lingering after-effects that prolong the recovery period. Depending on the method used, therapy may cause nausea, weight gain, skin problems, hot flashes and hair loss – sometimes more traumatic and harder to get over than the distortion or loss of a breast.

Things are busy at first, with many caregivers around to discuss problems and give advice, but as recovery proceeds there is more time to think about what happened. A woman may spend weeks or months recovering from the demands and after-effects of chemotherapy. She can feel very isolated without access to caregivers from whom to seek advice. Only after treatment is over do most really begin to face the emotional meaning of having cancer.

Try to Pamper Yourself during Recovery

The long period of therapy generally leaves women feeling weak and exhausted. Given the pervasive and debilitating after-effects of treatment, many despair of ever "getting back in shape," regaining arm movement, feeling strong enough to play tennis, swim, hike, jog or do all the things they did before. Recovery may be slower and take longer than expected. One oncologist suggests that women should allow themselves to feel lousy, and should look after and spoil themselves while recovering, letting family and friends take on the chores. "No need to be a hero or Superwoman all the time," he says. "Solicit help from friends, relatives, children, as well as formal support services available through the healthcare system." One counselor advises women to get rid of the "born to serve" mentality and ask others to serve them for a change. However, many women find this hard to do, having spent most of their lives as nurturers – caring for others rather than looking after themselves.

Getting Professional Advice

Accurate information about the recovery process and what to expect is a help in regaining a sense of control after the helplessness many feel during the treatments, what may seem like "assembly-line technological care." Some women leave their fate to the medical establishment, taking little responsibility for their recovery. But most try to take part in the healing process. However, finding one's way through the tangled web of the cancer care system and getting the needed advice is far from easy.

Although some physicians allot enough time to dealing with women's questions and uncertainties, others are not very patient, supportive or reassuring and are often not the best source of information. Other caregivers – such as psychologists, dietitians, specialized nurses attached to oncology units – can give more practical advice and reassurance, but also aren't always accessible. Physiotherapists can be extremely helpful not only in demonstrating exercises that speed recovery, but also in giving general image-improving and health advice, reassuring women that strength and abilities will return. Getting specialized counseling or sharing mutual experiences with others at a similar stage in the disease can also help women recover faster.

Getting the Body Back in Shape

Whether a woman has a lumpectomy or total mastectomy, if armpit nodes were removed, the muscles and other tissues of the chest wall, shoulder and arm will be affected, and often leave her with a stiff arm and shoulder that impede everyday tasks such as washing hair and doing up back zippers. The arm and shoulder may swell up. Some women develop "tethering" – attachment of the tissue under the skin to other tissues beneath – which feels as if tight cords under the arm are restricting movement and limiting the ability to lift the arm or straighten the elbow.

Physiotherapists can teach women exercises to restore arm mobility or, for example, demonstrate ways to relieve "frozen shoulder" or arm-swelling (lymphedema) – another frequent problem after breast cancer operations. Physiotherapists generally come around while women are still in hospital to teach specific arm movements, usually slow stretches, to avoid or release tethering, and suggest a set of exercises to be started as soon as possible after surgery. Physiotherapists can also help people regain a healthy sense of the body. If they don't come around, ask your family physician or other caregiver to refer you to one.

By the time women go home most can move their arm enough to brush their hair and do up zippers. Continuing daily arm exercises when home can reduce the discomfort and severity of *lymphedema* or fluid buildup. The best rule is "little and often," with the arm exercises done several times a day in short spells rather than one prolonged bout. Each woman must learn how much exercise and activity she can do while recovering; too much can trigger a muscle spasm or pain. Exercises with weights are gradually added until the shoulder can move normally and the muscles have recovered their strength. The best way to maintain full arm movement is to incorporate an appropriate exercise program into your daily schedule. Physiotherapists can help in answering questions about exercising or daily activities.

Resuming Normal Activities

- *Carrying things:* Shoulder bags and heavy handbags should be carried on the "good" side. Using backpacks or waist pouches can avoid arm and shoulder strain, but avoid uneven weight on the shoulders. Briefcases can be carried in the "good" hand, but shouldn't be too heavy. It's better to push, not pull, any heavy item, when using the arm on the operated side.
- *Ironing:* This is difficult because most of the movement is

produced by the pectoral and shoulder muscles; get someone else to iron or do it in short bouts.

- *Doing dishes:* Regular dish-washing isn't a problem, but scrubbing pots and pans requires care during the first few weeks after surgery. If still undergoing chemotherapy and radiation, limit any work that overexerts or strains the arm and shoulder on the operated side.
- *Gardening:* Sit on a stool and use hand tools to avoid overuse of shoulder and chest muscles (use a low stool to prevent back strain).
- *Avoid injuries on the operated side;* there's extra risk of infection if the lymph nodes were removed. Wear gardening gloves!
- *Lifting:* Don't lift or hold heavy items on the affected side.
- *Swimming:* Begin with a slow crawl. Gradually work up to more and faster lengths, but stay clear of breast stroke and butterfly during the recovery period as they put more load on the arms.
- *Tennis:* Begin with racquet exercises – bounce the ball on your racquet before really playing a game.
- *Aerobics (fitness) classes:* Start with low-impact classes, and go easy on arm exercises; step aerobics can give a good workout without too much strain on the arms and shoulders.
- *Golf:* Start gently; try putting first, then work up to the driving range.
- *Skiing downhill:* Be cautious. Don't ski on ice, hard pack or moguls to begin with. Ski deep powder last.
- *Skiing cross-country:* A support garment is advisable to reduce arm and shoulder overuse as it's very hard on the arms.
- *Weight training:* Use free weights and light hydraulic weights, and increase weight very gradually.
- *Boating and sailing:* Be cautious and wear a support garment

because of the arm strain these sports involve.

Controlling Lymphedema

Lymphedema, or fluid build-up and swelling in the arm due to removal of the lymph nodes and channels, can be awkward, persistent and painful. Normally, tissue fluid drains from the arm, through the lymph nodes in the armpit and back into the bloodstream. This flow is slowed down or blocked if some underarm lymph nodes are removed, or if scar tissue forms from radiotherapy. Fluid may accumulate and the arm may swell up. It's less common now that radical breast surgery is less frequently done, but still affects 10 percent of those having breast surgery, and is worsened by radiation therapy. It is usually mild and manageable with the right advice – which is not always available or given! If much underarm tissue has been removed, or the chest wall is affected, lymphedema can linger on or recur for many years, even indefinitely. It can be very severe in those with chest wall involvement; the arm may swell to a huge size, requiring special therapy.

Symptoms of lymphedema are arm swelling, a shoulder ache or a feeling like a tight band around the upper arm. It limits mobility and, in severe cases, impairs finger and nerve function. Occasionally the arm widens by 5 cm (2 inches) or more in circumference, and the trapped lymph may harden, leading to permanent changes in skin texture and color.

Unfortunately, many women endure persistent postsurgical arm swelling in the mistaken belief that little can be done to reduce it. Do *not* let the swelling go without medical attention. Early treatment is essential. Get a physiotherapist to show you exercises that can make the swelling go down. Early treatment can control it and restore normal arm function. Besides exercises, elevation of the affected limb can help the fluid drain.

Raise the swollen arm whenever possible – especially in bed at night, propping it on pillows; elastic bandaging can also help reduce the swelling.

Protection against Lymphedema and Other Arm Problems
Protect the swollen arm from knocks and scrapes; wear long-sleeved garments and gloves for household chores, gardening or heavy work and oven mitts when around the stove.

Try to avoid cuts, burns and insect bites on the affected side, especially during chemotherapy and in the post-therapy period (as the drugs suppress the immune system). If an injury does occur, clean and disinfect the wound at once; ask about the need for antibiotics.

Learn to recognize the signs of infection: redness, a sudden increase in pain or swelling. If you notice these signs consult a physician promptly.

Elevate the arm to help the fluid drain "downhill." Position the wrist and elbow higher than the shoulder. Think about the arm position from time to time during the day. For example, after you have been up and about for two hours, sit and elevate the arm for half an hour; if you're traveling, try to get a window seat on the affected side so it's easier to prop up your arm.

Pump therapy may be helpful for severe cases. The pump ("lymphopress machine") uses a special air-bag or sleeve that helps squeeze fluid from the hand and arm toward the body. The pressure can be varied to provide a massaging action that gradually moves the fluid toward the body.

Compression support garments can also help severe cases by providing pressure to keep the swelling down after a session of pump therapy. Some women wear support garments all the time, and others use them for sports or other activities that involve repetitive arm movements.

Ways to Avoid Lymphedema

- Exercise the arm and elevate it for a while each day.
- Wear garments with loose-fitting sleeves.
- Change the arm position frequently.
- Use an electric razor instead of a blade to shave under the arms, to avoid nicks that might become infected.
- Wear gloves for outdoor work and heavy chores.
- Apply sunblock and insect repellent when outside; bites and burns can become infected.
- Moisturize the affected arm several times a day.
- Protect the arm from overuse.
- Keep wounds on the arm and hand clean to prevent infection, and treat any that do occur with antibiotics (consult your physician).

Filling the Gap: Prostheses

After mastectomy, most women need a prosthesis – a false breast or "bra filler." In the first few weeks after surgery, while the scar is healing, they usually wear a light foam shape, often supplied by hospital staff or Reach to Recovery volunteers. They give women a soft, "fluffy" breast form made of cotton to wear temporarily in a bra. About four to six weeks after surgery, this is replaced by a permanent, molded silicone prosthesis of the right weight and shape to match the remaining breast. This feels much like a normal breast, and some have nipples crafted in, to look as natural as possible.

Breast prostheses are not "one-size-fits-all," and just picking one off the shelf isn't as good as getting one professionally fitted. A prosthesis should weigh about the same as the other breast, so it doesn't destabilize posture or make the woman feel lopsided. Traditional prostheses fit into a pocket in a specially designed bra. But a normal bra can also hold a prosthesis in place, if the bra is substantial and the breast shape isn't too large. A prosthesis may seem heavy at first, and takes some getting used to. If it's properly fitted it shouldn't shift about, or rub or irritate the skin; once it's in place, you should be able to forget it.

A recent innovation is a prosthesis that attaches to Velcro glued directly to the chest wall. Body heat activates the glue and the Velcro strips remain on the chest wall for a week to ten days. They can be pulled off like ordinary adhesive strips.

Mastectomy boutiques sell prostheses, along with specially designed bras and bathing suits. Some stores specialize in selling and fitting prostheses, and some have salespeople trained in fitting them who know the products available. Reach to Recovery volunteers, local cancer society offices or nurses at regional cancer centers should be able to suggest stores. Check whether the cost is covered by medicare or by your private health insurance. In Ontario, for example, the provincial program covers 75 percent of the cost of a prosthesis fitted by a licensed fitter; the remaining 25 percent may be covered by group or private insurance coverage. The forms can be obtained from a licensed fitter but require a physician's signature.

Follow-up Visits and Medical Checkups

After completing treatment for breast cancer, women are medically checked every two to six months, depending on the individual case, to monitor recovery and detect recurrences. Follow-up visits are most frequent during the first two years after diagnosis, tapering off later if there is no sign of recurrence. Breasts, chest wall and lymph nodes are carefully examined, as well as lungs, liver and abdomen.

Blood tests are done to check blood chemistry and look for tumor markers.

A bone and liver scan may be ordered, especially in high-risk cases or when there was evidence of spread.

No matter how good the recovery – despite signs that the

disease has been caught in time, even despite a reconstruction that returns the breast to a "normal look" – each visit to the doctor understandably engenders anxiety and is a grim reminder that the cancer may recur. Nonetheless, these check-ups are essential. Mention any significant new symptoms, such as persistent pain, or shortness of breath, nausea, weight loss, any new lumps or bumps. Don't overlook anything; ask about whatever worries you.

Facing the Stress of Breast Cancer

Breast cancer often engenders a crippling sense of defeat and helplessness, a shattered self-image, a sense of doom and of being unable to cope, even unable to tell anyone, let alone face the uncertainty ahead. To add to the stress, women sometimes feel upset by the way news of the cancer was delivered; their complaints may be justified, but there is no "good way" to tell someone she has cancer. Similarly, many are appalled by the impersonal, cold manner in which hospitals or clinics deliver the treatment, and the sometimes matching attitude of physicians. However, the medical system is not set up to guide people gently through the intricate technology, uncertainties and fears of treating this possibly lethal disease. Women must develop some way to withstand the clinical atmosphere and try not to be too stressed out or intimidated by it, especially as ongoing medical checkups are an essential part of recovery.

The emotions triggered by having and being treated for cancer typically include anger, a sense of being "picked on" and hostility. Some women worry that their thoughts and emotions are somehow abnormal, or an "overreaction," and that there must be a "better way" to respond or feel. Nothing could be farther from the truth; reactions typically span the full gamut of human emotions. They range from anger and anxiety to depression and helplessness – even feelings of guilt that one has somehow brought on the disease by wrongdoings, misdeeds or delays in going to the doctor. Many go through bouts of thinking they deserved the ill fate: "If only I'd eaten more sensibly," "drunk less alcohol," "been nicer to my husband [kids, mother]." The emotional roller-coaster can last several weeks or months – even years – going from disbelief to anger to denial, acceptance, then grief and perhaps profound depression.

Grieving over one's loss is a normal part of the recovery process. Those with breast cancer often hit a particularly vulnerable period about two to three months after treatment starts, frequently experiencing a series of reactions very similar to those that follow bereavement. There may be intense anxiety, with sleeplessness, loss of appetite and mood swings. Learning stress management techniques can be a great help.

Depression is common. It's marked by sleep changes, anxiety, feelings of shame and worthlessness – particularly if there are also changes in a woman's lifestyle or sexual relationships. (Often, women find it impossible even to look at their scar, let alone allow a lover, spouse, friends or family to see it.) Women need a great deal of support and reassurance about their continuing attractiveness and value during the stressful recovery period. Those who suffer deep (clinical) depression should seek expert advice and psychotherapy. They can ask for referral to a psychiatrist or other therapist. There *is* help available to combat depression.

Healing and Recovery Take Time

As the incision heals, the redness fades, the arm recovers its flexibility and the body regains strength, the soul and psyche also start to heal, although it can be a tough, slow road. Besides physical problems, breast cancer often triggers profound psychological changes that can affect lifestyle, relationships, work and goals. All of these aspects must be faced as women recover and take back their lives. They need someone with whom to share their worries, and on whose shoulder they can have a good cry. Those with young families will need extra support during the recovery period.

Family and friends are not necessarily the best people to offer reassurance, as they are dealing with their own fears about the situation – afraid of losing a wife, companion, mother or lover, and also facing their own mortality. Indeed, their concerns may come out as hostility or false optimism, which is not very helpful. They too need emotional support, to help them cope with their fears. (Counselors can help relatives, partners, spouses, children and companions of those with cancer who need emotional support.)

Gaining a Sense of Control or "Empowerment" Speeds Recovery
Regaining a sense of "wholeness" and personal control over the disease is critical to recovery. Many studies show that gaining what psychologists call "empowerment," or a greater sense of personal control, can enhance recovery from breast cancer and help overcome the feelings of helplessness. There are various ways to gain control. Some try to give their body a "fighting chance" by changing their lifestyle – giving up alcohol and cigarettes and adopting healthier eating habits. Many decide to "beat the cancer" by mind-over-body efforts and by changing psychological and spiritual attitudes. There is increasing evidence about the mind-body link, its effect on the immune system and the efficacy of psychological strategies in gaining a sense of mastery over illness.

In the past 30 years much research has shown that mind-body interventions play a key role in recovery from disease and has also shown the powerful impact of good doctor-patient relationships in assisting the healing process. But it's hard for women to be assertive, show a fighting spirit or gain control while recovering from the debilitating effects of cancer treatment.

Seeking information, turning to others in a similar situation for support, developing a partnership with the health-care team, maintaining hope and learning stress management techniques are all ways of developing a coping "mindset." Social workers, nurses attached to radiology or oncology units, dietitians, nurse practitioners, psychologists and psychotherapists can lend a sympathetic ear and give practical advice and are often better at explaining things than physicians. Nurses with special education and experience in cancer counseling can help women cope or guide them to valuable community resources. There are now many community organizations, such as the Breast Cancer Info Exchange Project, federally funded by Health Canada with branches across the country, and similar organizations in the United States. (See resource list at end of book.)

Support Groups Play an Increasing Role

Self-help or mutual-aid and support groups, survivor networks and activist organizations have become an integral part of modern breast cancer management. Some groups, such as Reach to Recovery and CanSurmount, put people with cancer in touch with each other, providing counseling, education and information. There's no need to wait for a referral from a physician or nurse. Any woman (or relative or friend) can call the cancer society to request a visit from one of their volunteers, if available, either during the hospital stay or while recovering. Their very presence as long-term survivors can give a woman more hope and courage than any words from someone who hasn't "been there."

Some organizations and survivor groups run self-help or peer support groups, most led by professional therapists or survivors with special training, some more or less political and led by "activists." They are a forum for sharing concerns with others experiencing similar feelings and problems. Support groups do not suit everyone recovering from cancer, but they can help people acquire stress-management and coping skills. They provide an opportunity to share emotions, to express anger and grief, and also allow members to bond with each other. Women should choose one with participants at a similar stage of illness – for example, newly diagnosed women should not join a group of women with metastatic disease. Self-help and support groups can have a powerful effect in helping women recover from breast cancer. Controversial evidence from one study suggests that participation in support groups considerably improved *survival* time in women with metastatic breast cancer. This U.S. study found that, of 83 women randomized to group counseling, self-hypnosis or standard care, those who received group support had a survival benefit. These results have been much scrutinized and criticized. A University of Toronto study is looking into the question. There is no doubt, however, that women who get plentiful support feel better and have a better quality of life than those not as well counseled or supported. (See resource list at end for support groups.)

However, support groups aren't the ultimate solution; not everyone with breast cancer wants to join, or will benefit from participating. It's a highly individual decision. Some prefer to seek individual therapy or counseling, or to share worries with a close friend or confidante. Most of today's cancer treatment centers offer counseling and psychotherapy to patients and their families. Ask your primary physician or caregiver how to access them if you need them. Some people seek greater control by self-healing techniques or through "alternative" therapies, including relaxation, massage, therapeutic touch (energy-transfer techniques), yoga, imagery, music or art therapy. Some find these nonconventional therapies very comforting. (See also Chapter 19 for alternative therapies.)

"Cautious Optimism" Is Often a Useful Approach

Although many people oscillate between despair and hope, "cautious" or "guarded" optimism can be an aid to recovery. "Try to keep up your spirits," advises one survivor. "Remember that many people who have breast cancer treated at an early stage live without recurrence for decades afterward." As a defense strategy, some women learn to distance themselves from the disease or think about the cancer in the past tense. Others find different ways to avoid thinking about the disease every waking moment, and to prevent it from dominating their lives. "The best way to manage the disease," suggests one survivor, "is to try to look beyond the unpleasant treatments to a stage when life can return to normal." Psychological or "mind-over-matter" strategies can have healing power if women try to retain hope, carry on with daily activities and lead as normal a life as possible, even if they are fully aware

---

Tips to Improve Optimism and Preserve Hope

- Remember that something can be done. Breast cancer is a blow, but it can be dealt with, and there is help out there. Try to find information and helping organizations.
- Although the treatment may drag on and drag you down, look beyond it to the time when life will be much as it was before the diagnosis.
- Things can return to normal once you get through the tedium and unpleasant effects of therapy – whether it's radiation, chemotherapy and/or hormone treatment.
- If distressed by the disfigurement of mastectomy, ask about the possibility of breast reconstruction.
- Although no one would choose to have breast cancer, it is not an inevitable death sentence; it can respond to treatment and even be cured.

of the possibility of recurrence. Most eventually arrive at a calmer period of acceptance that enables them to get on with life.

Remain Vigilant!

Women who've had breast cancer are urged to continue monthly self-examinations on both the operated and healthy sides. Any changes should be reported immediately. But do not panic; many breast changes are *not* recurrences. Many women develop some scarring (fibrosis) in a breast after surgery and radiotherapy, or thickening along the scar. Often it's difficult to know if the thickening is cancerous or not, and a biopsy and mammogram may be advised. Mammograms are recommended for the irradiated breast every 6 to 12 months afterward. Mammograms of the unaffected breast are usually performed once a year or so, depending on the woman's age and her individual case.

SIXTEEN

Coping with Recurrences

Finding a recurrent cancer is a devastating blow, shattering hopes that the original treatment was successful in banishing the disease. It is a searing experience to have to go through the same treatments again – more surgery, more courses of radiotherapy, chemotherapy and/or hormone treatments. The immediate reaction on diagnosis of a recurrence is most often dismay, terror, a feeling of being "one of the unlucky ones," and fear of "dying next week." But having a recurrence or finding a secondary doesn't mean instant death. Given the right care and good luck, people with metastatic cancer can live for several years, even many years, keeping it at bay as a chronic disease. Although *local* recurrences can be treated and cured with no diminution in overall survival time, a woman who has secondary or systemic spread through her body must face the likelihood of an eventually terminal illness, with the attendant emotional crisis.

While women who find a recurrence aren't likely to die tomorrow or next month, or necessarily within the next year or two, the recognition of a probably shortened lifespan gives many women a pressing need to examine and overhaul their lives, and set priorities for what they really want to do and accomplish in whatever time is left. "The chief downside," explains one woman who had a recent recurrence of breast cancer 11 years after diagnosis, and now lives with metastatic disease, "is that it's hard to live from day to day, not making any *very* long-term plans, say five or ten years hence. Otherwise, the treatment I get keeps me well and functioning most of the time."

What Signals That the Cancer's Come Back?

Recurrent cancer can appear locally, at or near the site of the original surgery, or as metastatic disease anywhere in the body. It may be a new primary (a tumor not related to the original one) but is most likely due to some breast tumor cells (or fragments of their DNA) that escaped and formed a secondary cancer elsewhere. The secondary cancer contains the same type of malignancy as the original tumor, and will often respond to similar therapy.

A *local recurrence* in the operated area – in what's left of the breast, or in the armpit, skin, chest wall or lymph nodes – may not reduce a woman's survival chances. But those with local recurrence after mastectomy may also have the disease elsewhere in the body.

Treatment for a local recurrence will be roughly similar to the first time. Lumpectomy may be done for a small tumor, mastectomy for a larger one. Radiation, hormone manipulation and chemotherapy may also be used – perhaps stronger than last time around. The choice of treatment depends on the previous therapy and the tumor make-up.

Systemic recurrence or metastasis occurs most often in the bones, liver, lungs, lymph nodes, brain and soft tissues. Although most recurrences happen between two and four years after the initial diagnosis, breast cancer may recur many years later. The risk of relapse depends on various factors such as whether the cancer was in situ (localized to a small area of the breast) or invasive.

Hormone treatments are often the first line of therapy for metastatic breast cancer. Progesterone-like drugs such as megestrol can be helpful, or high-dose medroxyprogesterone – as effective as tamoxifen but with worse side effects, including marked weight gain and vaginal bleeding in some. Androgens (male hormones) are also sometimes tried, such as fluoxymesterone, but its masculinizing effects (facial hair, voice-deepening) are a drawback. A new group of drugs called aromatic inhibitors may also be used (they block estrogen production). Taxol or taxotere (containing diacetyl baccitin) may be used. If it's at least two years after the initial treatment and there is no involvement of major organs, tamoxifen is a likely choice for older women with hormone-receptor–positive recurrences.

Signs of Systemic Recurrence

It is often hard to know whether aches and pains are just normal everyday twinges or symptoms of metastatic disease. It takes time for a woman to trust her body again once she's had breast cancer; the worry of systemic spread makes it hard to relax and forget. It's natural to imagine that every little ache or pain signals a recurrence. If a pain comes and goes in a day or two, it is not likely to be cancer and there's no need to worry. If it's persistent, have it checked out.

Systemic cancer recurrences are rarely "silent" – except for liver metastases, which often give no signal of their presence; or liver metastases may cause abdominal pain, weakness, nausea and extreme tiredness. Symptoms of metastases vary according to the organ(s) affected. For example, breast cancer that has invaded the bones will cause skeletal (bone) pain, and perhaps stress fractures (with the slightest pressure), while tumors in the lung may produce coughing and shortness of breath. In general, symptoms of recurrence are more persistent than normal body aches and pains, and gradually worsen. For example, while a normal backache brought on by opening the garage door may hurt for a day or two and then fade completely, metastatic bone disease in the spine will come on gradually, may come and go with activity, and may respond to painkillers but will not completely vanish. If you're worried about a symptom, especially if it's persistent or getting worse, see your physician or oncologist. If everything turns out to be normal and the symptoms continue to bother you, they may be due to some disorder other than cancer.

In contrast to local recurrence, which may be curable with further local therapy, there is not much advantage to early detection of metastatic disease since little can be done to prolong overall survival. So most physicians do not recommend innumerable X-rays, scans and unpleasant tests to find metastases. Many women feel alarmed if caregivers don't respond to recurrences with the same haste as before, and may feel "neglected," but in fact it may be for humanitarian reasons. However, people can survive for many years with metastatic cancer, perhaps keeping it under control with occasional radiation to the affected bone or other site, or with tamoxifen or some other not-too-toxic drugs. Radiation therapy is of major benefit in relieving pain from metastatic cancer in the nerves, bones, and elsewhere, and even a single treatment can sometimes bring dramatic relief. It may be used from time to time to enable people to continue an enjoyable life.

Take the case of Brenda, who had node-negative breast cancer at age 51 and developed a pain in her side four years after a lumpectomy. Suspecting a pulled muscle, she had an X-ray, which showed nothing "bad." But since the pain didn't really vanish, she had it rechecked six months later, and this time a bone scan revealed a "hot spot" in her rib which was treated with radiation. She also started on tamoxifen tablets. (She later stopped taking tamoxifen because it caused vision problems – a rare side effect.) Through the next three years Brenda occasionally had other "trouble spots" in her thigh, shoulder and pelvis, and each time received a course of radiotherapy. She felt well with this sporadic treatment for almost four years, but later also needed various forms of chemotherapy which kept the cancer under control, although one of the drugs caused heart problems and she had to cease taking it. Through it all, Brenda has carried on her life as a teacher and mother, continued with regular aquafit exercise, yoga classes, skiing and cycling, also going to the theater and attending art classes (which she calls "wonderful therapy"). She regularly attends massage, therapeutic touch, visualization and other healing sessions at her local Wellspring center, and became involved in founding a new breast cancer support and resource center. "It's not so much hope as keeping up your spirits and trying to make the best of every day" is what she says has helped her most. "Trying to normalize things and lead a regular life is a good idea," says Brenda to others in similar situations. "When you're down and feeling lousy, coddle and be good to yourself; when you feel okay, get out and do whatever you want to – play golf, swim, go to movies, see friends, travel, relax and make the best of every minute." She suggests that routine everyday activities can help people "hang on," and normalize life. She also tells women not to let physicians pressure them into "smiling through" all the time, as some of the treatments are "not exactly a joy-ride." Trying to concentrate on the fact that the treatments – some of them quite toxic and unpleasant, however "state of the art" – are helping you "takes a lot of effort and energy."

Dealing with recurrent cancer is a matter of weighing the toxicity and ravaging effects of treatment to "buy time" versus maintaining as pleasant a quality of life as possible and making the best of the time left. Even after diagnosis of a metastatic recurrence, the best treatment for a woman with no symptoms who feels quite well may be no treatment at all until symptoms occur, because in some cases the side effects of therapy are worse than the disease. While some people will pursue every treatment avenue available – including new and experimental agents – others prefer to "let the body decide" and enjoy whatever remains of life.

Treatment needs to be individually geared to a particular woman's biological make-up, emotional state, family setup, social network and personal wishes. One oncologist advises women who are feeling fine and active to "think carefully about putting themselves through toxic cell-kill treatments, rather than enjoying a reasonable quality of life, however long it lasts."

Treatment of Recurrent Cancer

Local Recurrence after Lumpectomy
The treatment for a local recurrence after a lumpectomy can be a repeat lumpectomy and radiation (if it wasn't given before) but is generally a total mastectomy, because there's no point removing the lump alone if the rest of the breast remains at risk of developing cancer, and radiation cannot usually be given a second time. When it's likely that the cancer has also spread, or will do so in the near future, systemic treatment such as chemotherapy or hormones may be added.

Local Recurrence after Mastectomy
Recurrence after mastectomy can affect the chest wall or lymph

glands in the armpit, above the collarbone or behind the breast-bone. The cancer is removed by surgery and systemic therapy follows as appropriate.

Distant Metastatic Spread
Patients with metastatic breast cancer usually receive varied treatments, including a mix of hormones, radiotherapy, chemotherapy, adequate pain management, psychological support and sometimes surgery.

No Need to Suffer Pain
Cancer pain often responds better than other types of chronic pain to medication, but paradoxically it may be undertreated despite the fact that the drugs that can control it are freely available and well understood. The World Health Organization regards cancer pain relief as a top priority. Studies conducted in the last decade show that too many physicians and nurses, as well as the general public, retain the outmoded idea that pain-killing drugs lead to addiction, or that it's a "sin" or a "shame" to resort to opioids because of their link to abuse and crime. In reality, *pain retards recovery,* as does the mistaken belief that it's better to "tough it out." The prevailing outlook of modern oncologists seems to be to "take whatever gets you through this – whether it's drugs, chocolate éclairs or a glass of wine." Any means of relief is encouraged by most oncologists and cancer experts these days, and many promote round-the-clock pain medication for those who need it.

Modern Pain Control Can Give Continuous Relief
Progress in pain control has evolved largely from improvements in cancer care that address both physical and emotional suffering. This is part of palliative care (which includes the care of incurable conditions). But physicians still sometimes

prescribe too little pain medication, perhaps through lack of pain-control knowledge or because of unfounded fears about addiction. Addiction is *not* a problem in terminal cancer.

In the past, pain medication was mainly prescribed PRN – "on demand" or when pain returned. Today's approach is to prescribe painkillers *around the clock,* tailoring doses to achieve continuous relief and prevent pain from surfacing rather than waiting to treat it after it reappears. Whatever its cause, chronic pain requires continuous *preventive* therapy instead of permitting anxiety about it to build to the point where patients and their families become distraught. Hitting pain early and keeping it down at all times helps to reduce the overall amount of drugs needed, reduces unwanted side effects and banishes the fear and anticipation that magnify its intensity. Cancer patients are now encouraged to gain personal control over pain, sometimes administering drug mixtures themselves in doses that never let pain break through. People often feel better when they participate in their own pain management.

Advances in pain management were pioneered by the British hospice movement, started within British hospitals during the early 1900s, which established humane principles for palliative care. In North America, the word "hospice" has been largely replaced by the term "palliative care unit." The hospice concept of total pain management – now accepted world-wide – addresses mental, social and spiritual as well as physical problems. It is based on an analgesic "ladder" system, using non-opioid painkillers first, followed by mild opioids such as codeine, then stronger ones.

Poppy derivatives (or their synthetic replacements) remain the mainstay of modern pain management; physicians use the term *opioid* instead of "narcotic," which may have negative connotations. Opioid drugs include natural poppy derivatives (such as opium, codeine, morphine and heroin) and synthetic substances, such as meperidine (Demerol), that mimic the properties of opium.

The opioids or *narcotics*, from the Greek *narkoun,* meaning "to numb," remain the world's most potent painkillers, ranging from the milder *codeine* to the strongest known analgesics: *morphine, hydromorphone* and *heroin* (now legal in Canada and the U.S. for pain treatment). Opioid drugs bind to brain receptors, blocking pain perception. Increasing doses usually bring greater relief. Most opioids can be given by mouth unless the patient is unable to swallow, in which case the drug can be given rectally, intravenously or sublingually (under the tongue). New long-acting, slow-release forms aid pain relief. For selected patients, a small pump can now continuously infuse tiny opioid doses under the skin, giving excellent relief with few complications. Rectal suppositories bring swift relief.

Reactions to opioids vary greatly. Some people remain active even if taking morphine or other opioids for years, while others feel drowsy and need a stimulant to remain alert. Oversedation is an occasional problem in those who wish to carry on as usual, but drowsiness usually wears off in a week or two.

Total pain relief may take a few days or weeks to achieve. Severe, persistent cancer pain usually demands opioid drugs. Finding the right dose may take time, with a "rescue dose" prescribed and kept on hand in case the pain breaks through. Co-*analgesics* (non-narcotic painkillers such as anti-inflammatories and antidepressants), given together with opioids, can enhance relief. If the usual regimen fails, epidural (spinal) or subcutaneous (under the skin) administration may work.

Addiction Is Not an Issue

Experts repeatedly stress that, although some physical dependence is usual after taking opioids for a long time, psychological dependence hardly ever occurs among pain patients. Requests for more medication from cancer patients generally represent disease progression and greater pain, not drug addiction. Cancer societies around the world emphasize that addiction to opioids among pain patients and those with incurable illness is *extremely rare*. One specialist points out that when pain patients are told to start on opioids, most accept reluctantly. "They have too much to do," adds one patient, "and don't want to be totally zonked out." Experience shows that, while some tolerance builds up in pain patients, it is usually predictable and the amount of medication needed to quench the pain soon stabilizes. If one medication doesn't work, another can be prescribed.

Opioid Side Effects Are Easily Banished

Side effects can be a problem with opioids and need to be prevented or treated as soon as people start on these painkillers. Stomach and digestive problems are especially troublesome. Constipation (which occurs in about 90 percent of patients) can be troubling and nausea (common in 60 percent of opioid users) gradually wears off, but experts suggest that, when prescribing opioids, healthcare givers should also routinely prescribe a laxative and antinauseant.

Constipation can be counteracted by a diet rich in fluids and fiber, the use of stool softeners and stimulant laxatives (in consultation with a physician).

Nausea and vomiting – common when people start to take opioids – usually disappear in a week or two. They can be offset by anti-emetic medications such as haloperidol, prochlorperazine, metoclopramide and domperidone. Dimenhydrinate

"Twilight Sedation" – an Occasional Last Resort

Most terminal patients can be kept reasonably pain-free. However, in an extremely small number of cases, when the disease is very advanced and pain cannot be well managed, some units employ "twilight sedation." This highly controversial procedure involves heavy sedation with an opioid plus tranquilizers, sometimes for weeks, until death. Twilight sleep has aroused concern among health professionals, some of whom believe that it resembles euthanasia (mercy killing). However, other experts feel that when, and only when, all other options have been exhausted, forcing cancer patients to endure excruciating pain in the last stage of their lives is needless cruelty. Since the person is not in a coma but can be awakened at any time, the use of twilight sleep is regarded by some as a humane alternative to euthanasia, but it is used only in exceptional cases and only by mutual consent of patient and physician.

(Gravol) is not considered useful for opioid-induced nausea.

Drowsiness, sedation, dizziness and confusion are common in the first three to seven days of opioid therapy but after about a week the brain adjusts to the drug, remaining alert while benefiting from the analgesic effects.

Respiratory failure is unlikely if opioid doses are slowly increased but may occur (in less than one percent of patients). It can be reversed by an antidote.

Commonly Used Painkilling Drugs for Cancer

ASA, highly effective for many forms of mild to moderate pain, has the great advantage of being non-sedating. ASA is increasingly used together with opioids to control the pain of bone and other cancers that don't respond to morphine alone.

Other non-narcotic drugs useful against some types of pain include acetaminophen, antipsychotics such as haloperidol and anti-inflammatories such as steroids or NSAIDs (non-steroidal anti-inflammatory drugs).

A Run-down of Opioid Drugs Used for Cancer Pain:

- *morphine:* the standard opium derivative against which the effectiveness of all others is measured, now available in a long-acting form giving 8 to 12 hours of pain relief;
- *hydromorphone:* a more soluble morphine derivative and the most soluble opioid known (as strong as, or stronger than, heroin), useful for providing a lot of drug in a little fluid. It can be given orally or rectally, or injected. (This drug, not available in Britain, has largely eliminated the need for heroin to control pain in the U.S. and Canada);
- *oxymorphone:* about the same strength as morphine, this can be taken as rectal suppositories or by injection, giving four-hour pain relief;
- *diamorphine* (heroin): widely used for cancer pain in the U.K. and U.S. but not in Canada, it gives slightly quicker-acting but shorter pain relief than morphine;
- *oxycodone:* a morphine derivative similar to codeine, easy to take as tablets – usually mixed with ASA or with acetaminophen;
- *methadone:* a synthetic morphine substitute, well absorbed by mouth, with a longer-lasting effect than morphine;
- *meperidine* and *anileridine:* synthetic morphine substitutes that relieve pain for four hours at best, more likely three hours only.

Co-Analgesics That Can Increase Opioid Pain Relief

Tricyclic antidepressants such as amitriptyline or imipramine can reinforce the effect of opioids. Besides helping to lift depression (common in pain patients), tricyclics also suppress pain and act as sedatives. Known to ease headache, low back pain and shingles pain, these drugs are especially useful in treating pain from malfunctioning or injured nerves.

Cortisone and its steroid relatives (anti-inflammatories) can alleviate pain due to nerve injury or inflammation. Besides their anti-inflammatory action, steroids also increase energy, appetite and strength, thereby improving overall well-being. But they cannot be used for very long without adverse side effects.

Anti-convulsants such as methotrimeprazine or carbamazepine may help to relieve nerve-root pain, but in a few people carbamazepine lowers the white blood cell and platelet count, a side effect that may be a problem.

SEVENTEEN

Breast Reconstruction

After mastectomy, women have several options for restoring a normal-looking breast – a pad (prosthesis) worn inside the bra, a synthetic breast implant or breast reconstruction using tissue from another part of the woman's own body. Breast reconstruction is becoming increasingly popular. Plastic surgery now gives excellent results, especially if the new breast is fashioned at the same time as the mastectomy – although this is not always possible.

The reconstruction can be done at the same time as breast removal (immediate reconstruction) – with the plastic surgeon working alongside the breast surgeon – or it can be done later, even many years after mastectomy. However, many surgical units cannot offer immediate reconstruction; they may not have on staff a plastic surgeon experienced in reconstruction, or may lack the facilities to allow two surgeons to work together during the mastectomy. The options can be discussed at the time of diagnosis, so women can think and plan ahead whether they want reconstruction, and when. Or they may like to take time thinking it over. (Yet many women say neither option was even mentioned.) Some treatment centers do not offer it. But women can ask around to find one that does, if they so wish.

Any woman contemplating breast reconstruction should have a full, frank discussion with the plastic surgeon, and get a complete rundown of the techniques available, their failings and advantages; she should also recognize that the results aren't entirely predictable. If going for simultaneous mastectomy and reconstruction, be sure to choose a unit well versed in this complex operation, which is pretty extensive surgery.

Who Can Have Breast Reconstruction?
Women who had a mastectomy in the past and are now unhappy with the appearance of their breasts can benefit from restorative surgery. Women who had "wide margin" or extensive lumpectomy, losing sufficient breast tissue to create an obvious hollow in the chest or a discrepancy with the other side, can often also opt for it. Women having mastectomies after a recurrence (following lumpectomies) can also benefit. Except for the unwell, most women are candidates for some kind of reconstructive procedure. Even women known to have widespread disease may still find that breast reconstruction can dramatically improve their quality of life for the remaining time.

The Advantages of Breast Restoration
In obliterating the visible deformity, plastic surgery lifts the constant physical reminder of cancer and its threat to life. It restores a woman's body image and sense of femininity, and may even change her lifestyle, eliminating the need to wear a prosthesis, or restrictions on the types of clothes, underwear and swimsuits that can be worn. To some women, keeping or restoring a breast makes a huge difference in terms of their self-

esteem, their feelings of being a "real woman" and sexually attractive. It can help to promote a sense of wellness and encourage a return to "normality"; it can also help family, friends and "significant others" come to terms with the fact that someone they love has a possibly life-threatening illness, without being forcibly reminded of it. Reconstruction does not affect the recovery from cancer or treatment options. It makes no difference to the outcome of surgery, radiotherapy, chemotherapy or hormone treatments.

Women who cannot have or make poor candidates for reconstructive surgery include those who are in ill health or not strong enough for the surgery, those with advanced cancers or very large tumors, those who have had chest-wall irradiation, heavy smokers, women on multiple medications, the very obese, those who have unrealistic expectations and people emotionally unfit to face extensive surgery.

Not Everyone Wants or Needs Reconstruction

Women vary widely in their wish for reconstruction, and the motivation to choose reconstruction depends on many factors. After considering all the options and weighing up their priorities, many women decide against it, or decide to "wait and see." A thorough discussion with the caregiver team is mandatory. The plastic surgeon will explain the choices, and also the option of doing nothing right now. One plastic surgeon emphasizes that "we don't treat the disease, we treat the woman as a person, trying to enhance her self-image. We can put right the disfigurement but cannot do anything to cure the cancer." It's often a good idea for women considering breast restoration to consult others who have had the operation, or to seek advice from breast cancer advocacy or support groups to make sure they're doing "the right thing."

Some women with high self-esteem and a good support

network don't feel any need for a new breast. One surgeon notes that, in his experience, "after the recommended wait, about half the women contemplating breast reconstruction decide against it, having come to terms with their disease, gotten used to living without a breast, feeling good about themselves and unwilling to face more surgery." Many women learn to live happily with only one breast, feeling quite at ease with a prosthesis (although in very large-breasted women the feeling of asymmetry can be a problem).They refuse to buy into the myth equating breasts with beauty or sex appeal. The brush with mortality has clarified their priorities, and heightened their awareness that a woman's attractiveness stems not so much from breasts as from innate qualities. Others are happy to be rid of the cancer for the moment, and nothing would induce them to face further surgery unless absolutely essential. While reconstruction may sound appealing, they just want to get on with their lives.

However, some women feel "less than whole" or "no longer feminine," and are desperately depressed at having to wear a prosthesis – a depression known as *post-mastectomy syndrome*. For them, reconstruction reinstates their body image, improving their quality of life.

Timing Breast Reconstruction: Now or Later?

Many surgeons restore the breast at the time of mastectomy, but others prefer to wait six months to two years so that the woman can think things over. The wait also permits the incision to heal and allows early local recurrences to be more easily detected. Reconstruction is usually delayed if radiation or chemotherapy, or both, are to be started immediately after surgery as these treatments can slow healing.

Breast reconstruction always takes second place to the main cancer therapies, and must be planned in a way that does not

The Benefits of Immediate Reconstruction

- There is less psychological trauma from loss of a breast.
- It avoids the need for two operations – having to face more surgery at a later date — and has better success rates.
- There's no need for a prosthesis.
- It eliminates restrictions in choice of underwear, swimsuits and other low-cut garments.
- It is less disruptive to a woman's self-image.
- The woman never has to see her body without a breast – she awakens from the anesthetic with a new breast.
- Immediate reconstruction need not interfere with chemotherapy or radiation as the scar will have healed by the time the therapy is started.

The Advantages of Delaying Reconstruction

- It avoids the longer, more extensive surgery involved in doing both at once.
- Some oncologists prefer to complete treatment before any breast replacement takes place.
- It allows oncologists to palpate the breast more easily when looking for recurrences.
- Some women who desperately seek reconstruction before they start cancer treatment no longer want it afterwards.

interfere with them. The *primary* goal in breast cancer treatment is curing or treating the cancer. Before the breast surgery is scheduled, women can seek assistance in going through the options so they can make a well-informed decision whether or not to have reconstruction – "now or later."

Women suitable for immediate reconstruction are those with cancers that don't involve the muscles and who are healthy enough to withstand a much more extensive and longer operation. Smokers, people who suffer from diabetes, those who take multiple medications, the very obese and sedentary and those with unrealistic expectations make poor candidates for immediate breast reconstruction.

Building a Breast from Body Tissues

Reconstructive self-tissue ("autologous") breast reconstruction has been available since the late 1960s, but at first it was a crude method with unsatisfying cosmetic results. Better surgical techniques have greatly improved the results, and self-tissue breast reconstruction is now widely done at more and more centers. There are several ways to construct the new breast, each with advantages and disadvantages.

The method of reconstruction depends largely on the woman's physique and the state of her chest. The "autologous" technique, which uses solely the woman's *own tissue,* is today's most recommended method. It takes muscle and skin from elsewhere in the body – usually from the lower abdomen – by a "tummy tuck" or *abdominal flap* operation. A flap is removed from the abdominal wall (from the "roll" or "spare tire" often seen when seated) and pulled up, or cut out and placed into, the defective chest area, providing the skin, fat, blood vessels and muscle for a new breast. (As an added advantage, it also flattens the tummy!) A new nipple may be created, using tissue from the unoperated breast (or other tissue flaps) and tattoo dyes to match the other breast. An alternative method uses tissue from the back to make a new breast.

The *transverse rectus abdominis myocutaneous (TRAM) flap* is becoming the most widely used method for breast replacement. The operation usually takes up to two hours, with a one-week hospital stay, but experienced teams do the operation in less than one and a half hours, with a three- to four-day hospital stay. A portion of skin and fat is taken from the lower abdomen, along with some muscle to provide a blood supply, and the "flap" is transferred to the chest wall to form a new breast mound.

TRAM (Transverse Rectus Abdominis Myocutaneous) Breast Reconstruction: "Tummy-Tuck Operation" Simultaneous with Mastectomy

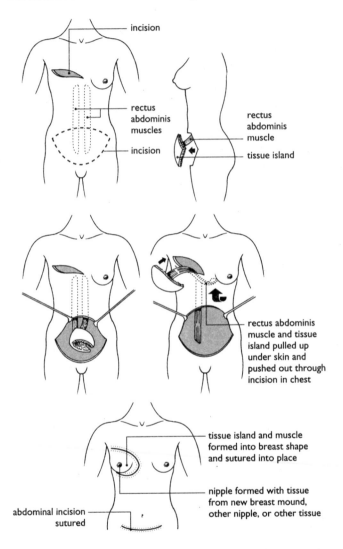

A patch ("flap") of abdominal skin and fat is isolated, along with some muscle to maintain a blood supply to this skin "island." The flap of muscle, skin, fat and blood vessels is placed in the breast area and shaped into a new breast mound, and the abdominal incision is closed. A nipple can later be formed out of tissue from the inner thigh, genital area or areola of the opposite healthy breast.

Other types of "free flaps" used in breast restoration include the gluteus muscle from the buttocks and the "Rubens" posterior flap which uses tissue from the hip.

Post-mastectomy breast reconstruction has advanced significantly in the past ten years. Refined methods can now create an amazingly natural-looking breast with a low rate of surgical complications (under 5 percent). The advantages over using implants are that there is no tissue rejection or reaction to a "foreign substance," and that it gives a softer, more natural look.

The main disadvantages of such restoration are the extensive surgery (with the usual complication rate) and a large additional scar across the abdomen or wherever the tissue is taken from.

The Tissue-Expansion Implant Method

A somewhat complicated option, particularly suitable for women with large breasts, is to insert a "balloon" under the chest-wall muscles and gradually inflate it with saline (sterile saltwater) through a valve implanted under the skin. The saline injections are usually done in the doctor's office. The injection

General Concerns about Implants

- They are less natural-looking than reconstruction from body tissues.
- They cannot be used if the skin is very thin, muscle has been removed or the area is heavily irradiated.
- They only give good results if used to fashion a small to medium breast.
- They may hinder detection of recurrent cancer in the reconstructed breast (a steadily diminishing risk as detection methods improve).
- There is a risk of allergic reactions to "foreign material."
- The body's reaction may cause hardening and give discomfort and a deformed look, requiring corrective operations.
- Rarely, leakage from the implant necessitates repeat surgery.
- They lack the erotic sensitivity of normal breast tissue.

port is a small plastic box that should not bother the woman at all during the months that it's in place, and injecting the fluid hurts no more than an immunization shot. It takes two to three months of saline shots, with 50 mL being injected every week or two, until the new breast mound matches the size of the opposite breast. This process gradually stretches the skin and surrounding tissues, and leads to a natural-looking breast shape. The bag may be removed and replaced with a permanent implant at a later date.

Breast Implants

Most breast implants used today are smooth-surfaced, saline-filled silicone balloons placed under the skin or muscle of the chest wall. Silicone-gel implants are no longer available in Canada owing to concerns about their safety and frequent leakage. In the U.S., silicone implants are under review. Saline implants may be smooth-surfaced or contoured and, under certain circumstances, silicone-gel implants are still permitted — for "charitable reasons." A new type of implant filler made of triglyceride with soya derivatives is already being used in Europe and is under clinical investigation in the U.S. Its great advantage is that X-rays can "see through it" and detect breast abnormalities that may be obscured by silicone-gel or saline-filled implants. Implants are useful in certain cases of breast restoration, especially in thin women with little tissue to spare. The implant can be inserted and filled at the time of mastectomy or later. Although most modern breast implants are safe, the body's normal reaction to foreign material forms scar tissue around them. Known as *capsular contracture*, the reaction may create a tough shell, giving the implant an unnaturally firm appearance, producing discomfort and sometimes disfigurement. The problem can be corrected by an operation that releases the contracture. However, the hardening may persist, and implants often require several adjustment operations.

Nipple and Areolar Reconstruction

Some women are perfectly satisfied just to have the shape and mound of a new breast to fill out bras and swimsuits and provide normal-looking cleavage. Others use plastic stick-on nipples to achieve the right breast contour. However, for the many who want it, a nipple can be made surgically after the main breast reconstruction has been done. It means yet another operation, since nipple reconstruction is best done after the reconstructed breast has settled for several months, so that the new nipple ends up in a position that matches the other side. The nipple construction is, however, only a minor "same day" operation. Both the nipple and the areola must be made using skin grafts from other parts of the body. "In practice," says one plastic surgeon, "the nipple is best constructed by sharing part of the areola from the opposite breast. It can also be done with a graft of a small part of the labia or skin from the inner thigh that has a darker coloration. A nipple may also be fashioned by using a small local skin flap that is bent like a caterpillar and the color then tattooed in. Tattooing is also the best way to make the areola, the darker skin that surrounds the nipple. Other ways of making the areola are by grafting part of the opposite one if it is large enough, or by grafting a thin slice of skin with tattoo pigments smeared under it."

In the hands of a skilled plastic surgeon, today's reconstructive methods can create a nearly normal-looking breast that almost exactly matches the other. Many women report great satisfaction with their reconstructed appearance. Those who had previous mastectomies and delayed reconstruction often also report a renewed self-image.

E I G H T E E N

Living with Breast Cancer

Having breast cancer is a major life crisis. While the initial reaction is devastation at the thought of losing a breast, that fear is later overridden by the realization of having a potentially fatal disease. Breast cancer no longer necessarily means loss of a breast, but no matter what kind of surgery or treatment women have, once they begin to recover, the threat of cancer can hit with a vengeance. Only after the treatment stage ends do most women begin to face the implications of having cancer. One psychiatrist who specializes in cancer management notes that "ultimately most women are more concerned about having cancer than losing a breast." Too few realize, she adds, that "there *is* a life after being diagnosed with breast cancer."

After the initial shock many women cope amazingly well, often tapping unexpected inner strengths that help them deal with the disease, accepting new realities, regaining a sense of control, finding ways to cope and live with breast cancer. Some even report a heightened enjoyment of life and better interpersonal relationships.

Adjusting to a Major Life Crisis

Although everyone with cancer must travel a unique path, there are some common features – alternating peaks of hope and despair, optimism and fear, and nagging uncertainty about the future. In coming to terms with cancer people typically experience preliminary shock and disbelief, denial, anger at being "singled out," unmerited self-blame for having brought on the disease (by unhealthy lifestyle, stress or other personal activities) and finally acceptance and resolve to "beat the cancer." Psychologists explain that these emotional swings protect against despair by allowing a "breathing space" for adjustment.

The jolt of having cancer makes people probe what they value and "who they are," rethink what's important to them and maybe alter their lives accordingly – sometimes in a big way! There's an inevitable period of adjustment to having cancer, sometimes long and hard. Those who have early-stage breast cancer face different problems from women with more advanced or recurrent forms. As the body's strength returns, everyday activities are resumed and women pick up the threads of their existence. Nothing is *entirely* the same again, but taking back control of one's body and one's life, being actively involved in managing the disease – becoming "empowered" – can greatly improve well-being.

Denial, distancing and avoidance (not thinking about cancer) are common defense mechanisms and can help to maintain emotional balance. People may comment that someone is "in denial" as though it were wrong or dangerous, whereas it's a natural survival mechanism that enables people to overcome helplessness, maintain hope and somehow carry on. However, these defenses are only healthy provided they don't interfere with getting appropriate treatment.

Combating the Sense of Aloneness

Many women go through "treatment-withdrawal anxiety" when the medical therapy ends, fearing that once treatment stops, the cancer will return. After working closely with the medical team, many feel left on their own and isolated. The caregivers (nurses, oncologists, radiotherapists, technicians) are no longer a daily part of life, and friends who were supportive at first may begin to drift off. That's when individual counselors and self-help or support groups can be particularly helpful in allowing women to express their anxiety, bolster their courage and share their concerns. Being "connected" to others in similar situations can help combat the sense of loneliness and help heal the body and spirit.

Strong support networks are crucial in coping with and surviving breast cancer. Those without a family or close companion must seek support elsewhere, and a counselor or therapist can be of great assistance in helping a woman overcome anxiety and get on with life. (To find a support group, consult hospital oncology units, cancer organizations, breast cancer survivor networks or local survivor groups; for an individual psychotherapist, seek referral from your family physician or other caregiver – see also the resource list at the end of this book.)

Sharing Worries with Others Can Help

Women usually find it best to disclose the fact that they have cancer themselves, according to their own needs and schedules. Confiding inner fears and hopes can help to overcome the anxiety, increase coping skills and improve well-being. In the long run, it is easier and healthier to share feelings than to conceal them. Studies have shown that having a close "confidante" – friend, neighbor, colleague, nurse – to confide in and discuss feelings with enhances well-being and may even prolong survival. But there are some people it may be best not to tell – for example, an unfriendly employer, "loose-lipped" associates, family members who are too old or frail, too young or too emotionally fragile, and might be unable to take the bad news.

A woman's cancer can deeply affect her partner and family. Other family members may fear they'll get the disease. Partners of women with breast cancer must address their own personal reactions to illness, hospitals and death. They may worry that she will be mutilated, lose all interest in sex, be weak, sickly, in pain or die. (Men may also have to face the disease in mothers, sisters and daughters.)

Dealing with Self-Image Problems

Women who have lumpectomies often exhibit less damage to their self-image than those who have mastectomies – less diminution in feelings of attractiveness and femininity, less self-consciousness or embarrassment about their appearance, greater comfort in talking about their illness and their sexual and other feelings. "However," explains one plastic surgeon who specializes in breast reconstruction, "self-image after breast surgery largely depends on how a woman felt about herself and her body before diagnosis. Those whose self-esteem was based primarily on external appearances are most shattered by the disfigurement Others, having accepted the risks of a potentially lethal disease, stop worrying about the loss of a breast or its distortion. They regard the altered body as a *secondary* concern, and focus more on fighting the cancer, soon forgetting or ignoring the breast's changed appearance."

Overcoming the "Sword of Damocles" Syndrome

Although most women outwardly seem to regain full confidence and vigor, and take up where they left off, things never completely revert to normal. There's the scar or lack of a breast to remind them, and even after lumpectomy the breast may have an altered shape and feel firmer (from scarring due to radiation therapy). "Knowledge of disease is ever-present somewhere in the back of one's mind," reports one woman who had breast cancer. "It's often the first thing I think about on waking up, although the thought fades as the day's activities take over." She finds ways to prevent the cancer from dominating her life – for example, consciously distancing herself and arranging a daily routine that stops her from dwelling on it. "I compliment myself for not thinking about it for an entire day (week, month)."

Most women manage to forget about the disease for increasingly long periods – at first just now and then, while cooking dinner or on the job – then for whole days, weeks, months at a time. The fear of recurrence gradually retreats with passing time but still lingers in some hidden recess of the mind, and hangs like the symbolic "Sword of Damocles" over all women who have had breast cancer. The fear can resurface and hit at odd moments – perhaps just before a checkup, or when kissing the children goodnight, triggering a flood of sadness at the thought of losing or abandoning them, or when planning some event a few years hence (which may never happen).

Anxiety and Depression Are Normal Phases

Some degree of depression is almost universal during and after the recovery phase; it can sneak up when least expected and may persist for many months. All women with breast cancer, those who have lumpectomies as well as those who lose a breast, naturally feel anxious. One study of women taking part in a clinical trial showed that those who had lumpectomy suffered as much depression as women who had mastectomy, possibly because their fear of recurrence was greater even though their psychosexual adjustment was possibly easier. In fact, breast *distortion* can be as hard to take as breast loss. The key is to get professional advice and therapy to alleviate depression (which can undermine health and impede recovery). "Ask for help when needed," suggests one psychiatrist. "Don't allow yourself to feel overburdened or struggle on alone when depressed." Typical signs of depression include sleep and appetite disturbances, persistent fatigue, lethargy, helplessness, slowed thinking, self-reproach and intense feelings of worthlessness. (For help in overcoming depression, request referral to a psychiatrist, an accredited psychotherapist or a counselor from your oncologist or other caregiver.)

Getting Back a Life and Gaining Control

In order to "beat" the disease and give themselves the best chance of survival, it is crucial for women to gain a sense of mastery over it, retain hope, remain positive, do everything they can to enhance their sense of well-being and lead as normal a life as possible. It helps to acquire accurate information and take an active part in managing the disease.

Some get back a life by looking into themselves and sorting out their priorities, deciding what they want to do and accomplish. Many women decide to change their lives – take up a fresh interest, learn a new skill, join a fitness club, work on relationships, try self-healing methods such as meditation, relaxation, massage – whatever comforts them and improves their well-being. Many decide to adopt healthier lifestyle habits – eat a more nutritious diet, exercise more, reduce stress and undertake other strategies that may offset the progress of cancer, or prevent it recurring or happening in the second breast.

Many turn to "alternative" or complementary, unconventional therapies such as visualization, imagery, hypnosis, biofeedback, therapeutic touch or herbal remedies. (See Chapter 19 for details of alternative therapies.)

"Hope for the Best, Prepare for the Worst"

Most experts endorse the benefits of a "fighting spirit" for those battling cancer, in order to protect them from despair and optimize survival chances. An optimistic outlook is crucial for people with any stage of cancer, giving them the strength to endure or surmount the disease. "Loss of hope slows recovery," explains one psychologist. "It undermines adjustment and leads to helplessness, which is an awful feeling."

Hope means different things to different people, and tends to change over time, depending on the stage of the disease. "Hope must be maintained," says one specialist, "to avoid depression, which makes people feel worthless and ready to give up." Bolstering hope takes many forms. One strategy is to focus on the present and what is immediately ahead, rather than on the more distant future or the past, neither of which can be changed.

A belief in the power of mind over matter has led to what some call the "heroic" approach in battling cancer. One University of Toronto psychologist describes the heroic stance as "based on the assumption that spiritual and psychological factors can influence, even arrest, the progress of cancer." This attitude can be heightened or dampened by the way others behave. Family members and friends should support the idea that hope is a good thing. Hope is not usually false optimism or fake reassurance; it's built on the premise that "better days, even better moments, can count." The best approach is to try to make the very best of whatever time is left.

On the other hand, *false hope* and an extreme belief in the curative powers of a "fighting spirit" can retard adjustment, especially if a woman dedicates every minute to vigorous self-healing efforts, rather than just relaxing and enjoying herself, or if it means abandoning medical treatments that might fend off the cancer. If there is too much emphasis on mind-power, it can impede the normal process of mourning one's loss, of "having a good cry." In addition, should the cancer come back it can produce a profound sense of failure and dejection, a sense of regret at not "taking the risk of dying seriously," not making the best use of the time left and accomplishing more. It can also be brutally alienating when family members crudely insist on maintaining an optimistic attitude when the patient is frightened and in despair, and wants only to be protected and shielded. Forced hope is *not* supportive.

Be Kind to Yourself

"Be gentle with yourself," suggests one cancer therapist. "Allow yourself to enjoy life and be who you are, do all the things you've always put off." But this advice is hard for women to follow, since they're socialized to nurture others, putting their own needs last. Many have trouble overcoming the tendency to give rather than receive, and find it hard to give themselves permission to pamper or take time for themselves – an important part of the healing process.

Loath to admit to weakness or to be served by others, despite the fatigue, sleep problems and anxieties that often linger after breast cancer treatment, many women resume full duties too soon. They may try to protect the family and bear the brunt alone, putting on a brave face. "Don't be too hard on yourself," counsels one therapist. "Carry on as best you can, but allow yourself moments of sadness, let yourself be waited on, treat yourself to a massage, hairdo, lunch with friends, whatever makes you feel good. Remember there's no need to be a brave soldier *all* the time." She tells women to do whatever they most desire – learn a new skill, visit the Grand Canyon, the Rockies, Paris or Bangkok.

Taking Up New Interests, Setting New Life Goals

With the impact of breast cancer comes a sudden realization of one's mortality, a sense that life isn't really never-ending. Many women report that having cancer is a "rude awakening" which forces them to re-evaluate "what life's all about" and set new goals. It can trigger fresh vigor and purpose in life, even start someone off on an exploratory track or stimulate a new career. Some decide to do something different and more self-fulfilling. "I learned to cherish each day, each week," says one survivor, "to enjoy the sunrise and make each day more meaningful." To her, that meant changing relationships, taking more time for *herself,* shifting responsibilities to others so she could take up a career in landscaping.

Some throw down the dishcloth and declare independence. One woman, dedicated to looking after her demanding husband and three teenage children, reports that once she recovered from the treatments she decided to completely "revamp her life." To her family's astonishment (and dismay!) she announced: "Sorry guys, I'm no longer going to be around to fulfill all your little wishes. Instead I'm going back to college to take my history degree, so you'll just have to learn to cook, do the laundry and generally take care of things."

Is There Sex after Breast Cancer?

Women, and their partners, often worry that having cancer will dampen sexual enjoyment. Sexual activity may be diminished by breast cancer. Fearing rejection or revulsion, some women refuse to let their partners see the scar. Some feel humiliated by the altered body image, which decreases their sexual desire. They may avoid sexual touching, which can make the fear a self-fulfilling prophecy. As well, the endless treatments can cause long-lasting fatigue, weakness and sleep disturbances that dampen sexual desire. Some hormonal and chemotherapy treatments halt menstruation and induce menopause, which can make intercourse uncomfortable due to vaginal dryness – sometimes remedied by vaginal creams or lubricants.

Partners may be unsure how to treat women with breast cancer. If they initiate sex, will it seem callous and insensitive? If they refrain, will it be seen as rejection and a sign that she's no longer desirable? Partners need to talk honestly with each other about sexuality and how the cancer may affect it. Those who have sex problems can get help from a qualified sex therapist. Both partners may need reassurance and encouragement.

Sex *can* be as good as before, or even better. Perhaps because it is tinged by the sadness of possible death, there can be a "letting go," an abandonment of petty concerns about appearance, less vanity and more passion and tenderness. After all, a woman's sensuality and sex appeal do not depend on breasts alone, but on her entire personality and who she is. Many say the relationship becomes more honest and caring. The majority of couples report an increase in physical intimacy (more cuddling, closeness, togetherness and affection) after breast cancer diagnosis, although they may have intercourse less often. One woman says her relationship became far more passionate after her mastectomy because her partner sensitively caressed both the healthy and scarred side, and for her part she became less self-conscious, enjoying sex more than before.

For those in a stable relationship, it can be an enormous help if the partner accompanies the woman to doctor visits – from diagnosis to follow-ups. What little research has been done in this area suggests that, while (like any major problem) cancer can further strain an already crumbling relationship, in a happy and stable union the stress of illness can actually cement the couple's bonds. One woman relates how her sex life improved after breast cancer, because she threw vanity to the winds and concentrated on making sex as much fun as possible for both her man and herself.

Starting or contemplating a new romance can pose interesting conundrums: when should a woman tell a potential sex partner about her mastectomy or breast scar? How should she broach the subject? Would it be best to do it in a matter-of-fact, casual manner during a stroll; or to discuss it at the dessert stage of a candlelit dinner? Each woman must wend her own way in this delicate matter.

What Do You Tell the Children?
Another question is what to tell children. There are no hard and fast rules. "In general," counsels one expert, "it's best to be honest with kids and use the word 'cancer' as they're bound to find out sooner or later – perhaps overhear a conversation or hear a friend or teacher casually mention it." It is worse to have "mother's illness" appear mysterious, something hidden and horrifying, than to talk about it openly and demystify it. As a rule of thumb, one psychologist suggests letting the child determine what he or she wants to know. "Answer honestly, including admitting you don't know, and do not try to convey more than a child asks for." The right way to tell children depends on their age and emotional vulnerability. With a young child, the approach might be, "Mummy's ill but the doctors can help." Children need to know that the illness is not their fault. Children who are angry at their mothers are apt to say, "I wish you were dead." When Mom suddenly has a serious illness, the child may think he or she is to blame. Children must be told that they did *not* cause the cancer by any thoughts, words, misdeeds, anger, dreams or wishes. They also need to have the changes Mother goes through (e.g., hair loss, fatigue)

spelled out ahead, so they are less frightening. It's often a good idea to let teachers, caregivers and daycare workers know about the cancer, so they can keep tabs on the child's reactions and intervene if necessary.

"Are My Daughters Also at Risk?"

The chilling thought that a woman's breast cancer may also endanger her daughters often produces a dark cloud of worry and guilt. If the breast cancer is an isolated or first case in the family, it is likely to be a sporadic cancer that's not inherited; only about 4 to 6 percent of all breast cancers are due to known cancer-susceptibility genes. When there is an identified family risk, genetic counseling and family therapy, with close relatives (who may also be feeling frightened), can help. Many daughters and sisters react to the diagnosis of cancer in their relative with terror and become hypervigilant in checking for signs of it. Adolescent daughters in particular seem to react strongly, in an adverse way that can undermine their self-image and interfere with early sexual encounters. It's best to talk things out and work through the complex feelings. (In some families prone to breast cancer, the men are also at risk; see Chapter 11.)

Can Stress Bring the Cancer Back?

While stress can affect the immune system, and could conceivably undermine the body's ability to destroy cancer cells, scientific studies on the link between stress and cancer are conflicting. Some suggest that stress may be a contributing factor; others do not. While some authors, activists and "alternative" therapists claim that stress triggers cancer, there is no scientific validity to the idea that women "give themselves" breast cancer – and making them feel guilty about something they didn't bring about interferes with recovery. Self-blame is a real hindrance to healing, and women may need expert therapy to combat the unmerited self-blame. It can be especially destructive for women from abusive backgrounds who already have a "blame the victim" mentality, and are all too ready to shoulder the blame for having cancer or any other affliction that's in no way their fault.

Battling cancer with the accompanying uncertainty, the need to live "one day at a time," is undoubtedly stressful. And finding ways to reduce the stress with stress-management strategies such as music therapy and relaxation techniques can speed recovery. Research shows that even 20 minutes of relaxation each day has physiological benefits, no matter whether it's transcendental meditation, massage therapy or simply sitting quietly watching the birds or listening to music.

Can Diet Help?

Women with breast cancer often wonder whether altering their eating patterns can quench the cancer, extend survival and prevent cancer in the opposite breast or elsewhere. Most physicians say it's uncertain. But there is evidence linking high-fat diets to cancer, and some preliminary indications that diets low in fat (especially saturated or animal fat) may reduce cancer risks. Basically, diets that may ward off cancer are low in fat, and rich in fruit and vegetables. (Some studies also suggest that soya products and certain oils, especially flaxseed and olive oil, *may* reduce breast cancer risks.)

After breast cancer, women are generally advised to eat a well-balanced diet, following national nutritional guidelines. That doesn't mean rigid dietary rules, but rather choosing a variety of foods while still enjoying the pleasures of eating well. Specialized cancer-wise dietitians can be a great help in choosing a body-strengthening diet.

A good anti-cancer diet is basically low in fats – fat making up no more than 25 percent of total calories – with plentiful fruit, vegetables and whole-grain products, especially those high in beta carotene, vitamins C and E and other antioxidants. Basically, people should include 5 to 10 servings a day of varied fresh fruit and veggies in their diet. Adopting a healthy diet does *not* mean banishing all appealing or snack foods. It simply means changing the focus – for example, enjoying a bowl of whole-grain cereal instead of a doughnut for breakfast, or having fresh fruit for dessert more often than cake or pastry. If a woman finds it difficult to eat a variety of vegetables, fruits and whole-grain foods, a daily multivitamin and mineral tablet may be recommended.

Be wary of "alternative" diet therapies that include extreme or unbalanced diets – for instance, multiple servings of carrots a day (which can turn you orange), macrobiotic regimes or massive doses of megavitamins. Most extreme or fad diets have no proven scientific basis or life-prolonging value, and some are harmful. (See chapters 19 and 20.)

What about Pregnancy after Breast Cancer?

Becoming pregnant when there is already a cancer in the breast can speed up its growth, probably due to hormonal influences. But studies suggest that, a year or two after removal of a breast tumor – provided there has been no recurrence – a woman can bear children with no greater risks than usual.

Linking Up with Activist or Survivor Movements

Many women find that participating in survivor or activist groups – to help others and carve out better management for the disease – can be of great therapeutic benefit in coping with the illness. Breast cancer survivor networks and support groups have sprung up across North America to inform women, offer peer support, raise awareness, circulate newsletters and run self-help groups; some are also involved in activism. Breast cancer advocacy groups began to emerge in the 1990s to support and help women with breast cancer. They took an active part in the 1993 National Forum on Breast Cancer in Montreal, where for the first time patients with breast cancer joined health professionals, researchers and government representatives in scientific sessions and discussions, greatly enhancing the public image of the survivor and activist movement.

Survivor and support groups are for individual women, to help them share grief and empower them in coping with the disease. Those who take part often become "informed consumers," better able to manage their disease. While survivor groups concentrate on informing and helping individual women, advocacy and activist groups focus more on the collective needs of those with breast cancer. Activist organizations are more confrontational, and aim to provide a voice for women with breast cancer, raise consciousness, push for more media attention, publicize pressing issues and demand a greater part in the decision-making process. They want "meaningful participation in all levels of cancer research, and especially in finding ways to fill the knowledge gaps," pleading for more attention to cancer prevention.

Women with breast cancer – or their friends and relatives – who would like to link up with survivor or activist organizations can inquire at their local cancer society chapter, or contact breast cancer survivor networks or other cancer information projects, or support and resource centers. (See resource list at end of book.)

End-of-Life Choices
Sadly, there is no cure for those with advanced metastatic breast cancer. For them, palliative and supportive care are the

chief aim. Some will pursue any treatment or experimental drug going, to "buy time" at any cost, while others refuse toxic treatments, forgoing the dubious benefits in favor of enjoying whatever precious time is left. The choice is very personal. It can be a wise idea not to undergo toxic therapy but to stay relatively well as long as possible.

Women with metastatic cancer need pain relief, support, and lots of tender loving care. Many people find it agonizingly difficult to know what to say to someone with terminal cancer. Death and dying are no longer part of everyday life in the way they were to our forebears, when extended families lived together and most people died at home. Western society is a "death-denying" culture and many can hardly utter words like "cancer" or talk about death. Death has been a largely taboo topic, only now regaining the light with recent public discussions about euthanasia and doctor-assisted suicide.

Sometimes people feel that their relative or friend is best shielded from the knowledge that a disease is terminal, although studies repeatedly show that most people want to know the truth so they can complete "unfinished business," organize their affairs and perhaps repair broken relationships. People need honest information so that they can take care of personal, financial and legal business. They have "end of life" choices to make, for which many welcome assistance. Some wish to write "living wills," complete consent forms or arrange power of attorney to make sure their wishes for terminal care, life-support systems and funeral arrangements are carried out. They may want to be in touch with their spiritual advisors.

Understandably, none of this is easy if everyone else is avoiding the subject in embarrassment. People with cancer who are not told the truth often feel lonely, rejected and isolated, and seem to suffer more depression and anxiety than those who face the worst. Sometimes friends and relatives are terrified of referring to the disease at all, and it becomes an unmentionable subject despite the fact that it's the main topic on everyone's mind, silently dominating all interactions, creating an undercurrent of tension and awkwardness. In many instances the people with cancer *do* know, but join in the conspiracy of denial to avoid upsetting their relatives; indeed, sometimes "shielding" the sufferer is really an excuse for others to avoid facing the issue. Anyone who asks for the truth should be given it. People with cancer often want to talk about their feelings. Family and friends can be a great help by sensitively listening, just "being there" and not feeling a necessity to say anything.

NINETEEN

Alternative or Unconventional Therapies

In their search for relief, many people with cancer turn to "alternative" medicine – also called "complementary" or unconventional medicine. Disillusionment and waning confidence in the medical system are leading more and more people with chronic ailments such as arthritis or cancer to seek help from unconventional therapies such as acupuncture, naturopathy, homeopathy, visualization, massage or relaxation therapy. Both traditional physicians and most of those who practice complementary medicine believe that alternative therapies work *best* alongside or as a supplement to conventional treatment.

Although a few people use alternative therapy *instead* of suggested medical treatment – like those who give up their prescribed medication and go to Europe or Mexico for treatments not available here – most cancer patients wisely use alternative therapy not to replace medical treatment but in addition to it. Those who think of trying unorthodox therapies should do a thorough investigation of any alternative healing methods being considered. Ask your caregivers whether they might conflict with the medical treatment you are receiving.

Alternative Therapies Gaining in Popularity

In the past, some alternative therapies – typically described as "holistic," "natural" or "nontoxic" by advocates – were labeled by disapproving medical opponents as "dubious at best," perhaps even "outright quackery" or "fraud," and often considered potentially harmful – possibly even life-threatening. But some tenets of naturopathic and other forms of unconventional therapy are now gaining credence among conventional practitioners, and are no longer considered entirely "fringe" medicine. Physician attitudes are becoming less disdainful and some medical caregivers endorse certain non-mainstream therapies for use alongside standard medical treatment.

Provided they do no harm, unconventional therapies need not really be an "alternative" to standard therapy; many can easily go hand in hand with medical treatment. For instance, some cancer patients add massage therapy, yoga classes or herbal remedies to their physician-prescribed regimens. These complementary treatments are especially useful in giving people with cancer a greater sense of control over their lives, a feeling that they're "doing something positive," helping to maintain hope and optimism – which in turn may speed recovery.

Even when it is of no proven benefit or does nothing to halt the disease, unconventional therapy often improves the patient's sense of well-being and quality of life. In giving people comfort and hope some alternative healing methods strengthen the "fighting spirit" and can decrease disease symptoms. As well, unconventional healers tend to give more time and individual attention to their patients than most mainstream medical caregivers, and may thereby enhance the person's psychological and spiritual well-being.

In contrast to conventional medicine, which tends to standardize treatment according to broad categories, alternative therapies are often more individualized and "client-oriented." Also, the personal attention given by some alternative therapists can help overcome the helplessness that many people experience when undergoing technological medical treatments – such as radiation or chemotherapy – some of which are upsetting and conducted in cold, clinical surroundings. Many alternative healing methods also aim to stimulate the person's own recuperative powers, and make use of mind-body interactions and the fact that mental and physical health are closely interwoven.

There is growing recognition among medical practitioners of a need to examine how alternative treatments may augment or interact with mainstream treatments – and of a need for properly conducted trials to evaluate the effectiveness of some widely used complementary therapies. In response to public pressure, the U.S. Congress has recently established an Office of Alternative Medicine in the National Institutes of Health to evaluate alternative treatments that might offer promise in treating cancer and other disorders.

What Are "Alternative" Therapies?

Through the ages, thousands of alternative cancer therapies have been tried, ranging from the bizarre but benign – such as foot massage or reflexology – to the borderline conventional – such as exercise or relaxation therapy – to the out-and-out dangerous, such as coffee enemas, which can cause electrolyte imbalances and death. The cost of alternative therapies also varies widely, depending on whether cancer sufferers go to

$5,000-a-week laetrile clinics in California and Mexico or just drink exotic herbal teas.

Unorthodox forms of cancer treatment include a large number of so-called "unproven methods" – a catch-all phrase that covers therapies from megavitamins and "therapeutic touch" to immune stimulants and "metabolic" strategies. Unconventional remedies are often called "unproven" because they have not been subjected to rigorous scientific testing and scrutiny.

The many individual testimonials and personal anecdotes claiming improvement from alternative therapies do not provide solid scientific evidence for their therapeutic value, and outcomes haven't been objectively documented. This is not to say that the treatments have no validity, but most physicians feel uncomfortable about recommending or placing faith in an unconventional remedy without enough objective evidence to support its use. Much remains unknown about the adverse side effects of alternative treatments – and even herbal preparations can have severe side effects. In order to make an informed decision about any treatment, the person must have as much information as possible about the risks versus the benefits. In the case of standard treatments, the facts may be discouraging but at least they are known. In the case of untested, unproven remedies, there is no evidence to evaluate.

Another often criticized aspect of unconventional therapies is the secrecy that sometimes surrounds them. Alternative therapists may try to persuade patients not to discuss their complementary treatment with their physicians. Secrecy is unscientific; medicine progresses by shared information, discussion, replication of results, criticism and controversy. This is especially intense in the field of cancer, where research findings are made public so that disagreements can be aired and understood. It must be acknowledged, however, that much healing occurs outside the realm of medical science, and that psychological influences play a key role in recovery and health.

Who Uses Alternative Therapies, and Why?

An estimated 30 to 60 percent of people with advanced (metastatic) cancer participate in some form of alternative therapy. In Canada, the 1993 National Forum on Breast Cancer Survey found that 36 percent of women with breast cancer had used some form of "unconventional therapy."

According to figures from the Harvard School of Medicine, about 60 million North Americans have used some form of so-called alternative therapy in the 1990s. In fact, North Americans seem to make more visits per year to alternative practitioners than to primary-care physicians (425 million visits to alternative healers versus 388 million to medical practitioners). According to the U.S. National Institutes of Health, in 1990 Americans spent an estimated $13.7 billion on unconventional therapies, of which $10 billion was paid out of pocket, not by insurance plans – and these therapies are growing in popularity as the public becomes increasingly frustrated with conventional medicine.

Some reasons for the popularity of nonconventional therapies are that they are generally non-technological and person-centered, and that they appear less toxic and more "natural" than orthodox treatments, giving people a greater sense of mastery in directing their own care. This positive approach can help sustain hope and psychological health in facing the ordeal of cancer.

Other reasons why people turn to unorthodox therapies include the nature of cancer itself, and the failure of conventional medicine to help them. In the case of breast cancer, medical science has little to offer in the way of certain cure. If there is no effective medical treatment, many patients, especially those with advanced or metastatic cancer, will understandably seek help wherever they can. Also, some complementary therapies claim to boost the immune system and attack the cancer in a "natural" way, in sharp contrast to the high-tech solutions and drug treatments of conventional medicine. Many patients find holistic and natural programs gentler, less invasive, more individualized and more appealing than the toxic cell-kill of current medical cancer care.

Alternative Therapies Need More Scientific Scrutiny

Many conventional treatments for cancer have undergone rigorous testing for side effects versus benefits. The surgery, chemotherapy and radiation treatments given for breast cancer, for example, have been studied and documented in peer-reviewed scientific journals, according to strict scientific criteria, so their dangers are known and their possible benefits have been quantified. In contrast, most alternative therapies have not been scientifically assessed.

What Are Some Alternative Cancer Therapies?

The most common unconventional therapies fall into the following groups: metabolic or "detoxifying" efforts; special diets and megavitamin therapy; herbal therapies; biological and physical remedies (such as ozone therapy); homeopathy; immune therapy; acupuncture; and psychological, behavioral and imagery methods. Most alternative therapies claim to be useful for any type of cancer.

Patients may be offered a combination of treatments. For instance, the Gerson Institute in Tijuana, Mexico, offers a hodgepodge of liver extracts, coffee enemas, vegetable-juice diets, oxygen or ozone therapies, clay packs, live cell therapy and various vaccines. A therapy may have been invented recently or it may have traditional or religious underpinnings stemming from Native American or Chinese medicine. It may have a quasi-philosophical basis, such as the anthroposophy of Rudolph Steiner, or homeopathy's doctrine of "like cures like." Such approaches involve ideas of physical process that differ greatly from the tenets of Western science. The patient may be told about "bioforces," "energy meridians," oxygenation systems, magnetism and detoxifying remedies.

Metabolic Therapies

The theory behind metabolic therapies is that toxins in the body collect and promote cancer and that certain "cleansing" and "purifying" agents can detoxify the body. Many metabolic therapies are built around specific detoxifying agents such as *laetrile, iscador* and *hydrazine*. Laetrile, a drug made from apricot pits, was tested in a large study run by the U.S. National Cancer Institute which failed to show that it was beneficial. As well, there have been some laetrile-related deaths, possibly due to the cyanide that is an active component of apricot pits. The metabolic treatments using iscador (made from mistletoe) and hydrazine have not been studied so it's impossible to assess their risks or benefits. Other "cancer-curing" drugs (of no proven benefit) include antineoplastons, benzaldehyde, cancell and those used for "chelation therapy." (Physicians warn that chelation therapy can reduce the body's zinc levels and also deplete the blood calcium, with possibly serious consequences.) Antineoplastons supposedly "normalize" cancer cells but several people have died from their use.

Anti-cancer Diets

Too much animal fat is suspected of promoting the development of certain cancers, including bowel and breast cancer. Although there is mounting evidence that a high-fiber, low-fat diet can decrease the risks of *developing* cancer, no study has ever definitively proven that any type of diet cures or modifies the *progression* of the disease. Nevertheless, anti-cancer diets are popular. Some alternative anti-cancer diets are quite rigorous, involving elimination of certain foods, or fasting and purging. The "grape diet," for example, has the dieter eat nothing but "cleansing grapes" for weeks; the weakness felt is attributed to "dying cancer cells." Other unusual diets include *Kelley's diet* of raw meat and meat juice, the *macrobiotic diet* of grains and rice and the raw food cure. Many unconventional anti-cancer diets have been strongly criticized, not only because there is no evidence that they work, but because they may cause severe nutritional imbalances that increase the weakness of people already debilitated by cancer. In addition, the diets may be unpalatable and indigestible. For example, strict vegetarian macrobiotic diets of brown rice and cereals with very little liquid are too difficult for cancer patients to manage, and can be harmful as many patients are already losing weight and have poor appetites. Most physicians agree that good nutrition should continue during recovery from cancer, and suggest eating plenty of fruits and vegetables, lowering fat intake and increasing fiber as commonsense *recommendations,* but not as a cure. (For a diet that may help prevent cancer, see Chapter 20.)

Physical Therapies

A wide range of physical therapies are promoted for cancer patients, some involving electricity, radio waves, magnetism and oxygen. The oxygen is often administered as ozone (O_3), or as germanium sesquioxide, a highly active form of oxygen; or some of the person's blood can be passed through an ozonizer and then reinjected into the body. Ozone therapy, very popular in Europe and used by thousands, is based on the premise that cancer cells have different metabolic needs than normal cells, and prefer a "low oxygen" milieu. Promoters of ozone therapy believe that saturating the cells with oxygen provides a metabolic environment that is hostile to cancer cells. This therapy is widely used but can have some serious side effects, so it should be supervised by a well-trained practitioner.

Immune Augmentation Therapy

These treatments are based on the theory that cancer is due to an immune-system defect, and that if the immune system can be stimulated, the cancer may be controlled. For example, patients may be injected with *"lymphokine activated killer (LAK) cells,"* or heat-shock proteins (recently produced by genetic engineering, and said to stop tumors developing). The safety of some immune injections has been questioned – especially *live cell therapy,* in which fetal cells from animals (such as sheep) that tend not to get cancer are injected into humans, and can provoke allergic reactions, even cause death. *Burton's immunoaugmentive therapy,* carried out in a clinic in the Bahamas, involves injections of blood products, samples of which have reportedly been found to be contaminated with HIV (AIDS) and hepatitis viruses.

Although some cancers may be influenced by immune system function, others arise without any obvious connection to the immune system, and much remains to be learned about the link. Researchers and immunologists are struggling to determine what role the immune system plays in the development and treatment of various cancers. At this time, despite years of research, there are many unanswered questions, and although vaccines and medications to boost the immune system may have some validity, no such treatment has been proven to work against breast cancer.

Herbal Remedies

Herbalism, which originated from traditional Chinese medicine, is an ancient form of treatment using plant and animal extracts (often as pills or capsules). Herbs may be mixed in specific proportions to relieve pain, remedy heart ailments, treat cancer or cure other problems. Many modern medications derive from plants, although the healing ingredients are now often chemically synthesized. The heart drug *digitalis*, for instance, comes from foxglove plants; *morphine* comes from the poppy; *quinine* for malaria is made from cinchona bark; the chemotherapy drugs *vincristine* and *vinblastine* come from the periwinkle plant. Although most herbal remedies haven't been evaluated according to Western scientific standards, some have been extensively studied by equivalent methods. Many people are firm believers in herbal remedies (recently termed phytomedicines to denote their plant origins) and turn to them because the medical system fails them. Herbal remedies are available in health food shops, from traditional ethnic stores or from naturopaths and herbalists. Their regulation varies greatly from place to place. In some countries herbs are listed as medications, in others they are classified as foods. Most occupy a "gray area" between medications and food. In the belief that "natural" equals "safe," some people take herbs in huge amounts; but while most herbs are harmless when used in moderation, large doses of some (for instance, comfrey and gordolobos) can cause adverse reactions such as bleeding, gastrointestinal problems and liver disorders.

Psychological and Behavioral Therapies

Imagery, visualization, hypnotism, psychotherapy, psychological counseling and other psychobehavioral therapies have been widely promoted for cancer therapy, either alone or alongside conventional therapy. These therapies aim to reduce stress and alleviate depression, helping people combat disease. Dr. Bernie Siegel, a U.S. physician and author, claims that a "positive attitude aids healing and may even prolong life." One famous technique is *Simonton's technique* of "guided imagery," where the patient imagines his or her cancer as, for example, a weak crumbly thing, and the body's immune system as a strong force fighting it. The concept of "visualization" is that mental energy can be focused to destroy cancer cells or stop their growth. Relaxation and meditation therapy rely on the premise that a healthy mental attitude can aid healing.

Other methods such as massage therapy, "therapeutic touch" and other touch techniques also rely on a connection between mental and physical health. While these therapies have not been proven to work on their own, they promote a sense of responsibility and control that can reinforce other healing remedies. They are promoted by conventional therapists to improve the quality of life and to alleviate the stress of cancer.

Deciding about Alternative Therapy

Cancer societies and oncologists advise women *not* to abandon conventional therapy in order to pursue unorthodox treatments. No alternative therapy has ever been proven effective in curing cancer or in modifying the course of the disease. In addition, unconventional remedies may delay or replace standard therapy, reducing the chance of arresting early disease, or palliating the symptoms of advanced cancer. However, when used alongside–*not instead of* – conventional treatment, many unconventional therapies, such as relaxation, meditation, imagery, yoga, massage and psychotherapy, usually do no harm, and can be of great benefit in helping patients come to terms with their illness and gain a sense of empowerment with which to fight it.

In making the decision, it's wise to gather all the relevant information and weigh the risks and benefits. Some therapies are extremely expensive, running into thousands of dollars, and some are dangerous or highly unpleasant. People must take care to avoid fraudulent, harmful or excessively costly forms of alternative therapy, especially as some proponents or practitioners may play on the hopes and fears of ill people for monetary gain. Some questionable treatments that concern many cancer agencies include antineoplastons, cancell, immunoaugmentive therapy, laetrile and macrobiotic diets.

Discussing the planned therapy with a physician may assist in making an informed decision. Anyone going on an "alternative" or extreme diet or herbal medicine should tell the medical team, as some substances or regimes may interact unfavorably with conventional therapies. Two books that may be helpful to those interested in alternative medicine are *A Guide to Unconventional Cancer Therapies* (published by the Ontario Breast Cancer Information Exchange Project), which describes alternative therapies without endorsing any particular one, and points out possibly dangerous side effects; and *Alternative Medicine: Expanding Medical Horizons, A Report to the National Institutes of Health.* (See resource list at end of book.)

What Are the Risks of Alternative Treatments?

The risk of unproven or nontraditional therapies relates mainly to the lack of scientific evaluation and safety standards. We have no safe regulations for alternative cancer treatments. As well, the costs can be prohibitive. A therapy that promises a "cure" can make people with cancer willing to pay large sums of money regardless of the lack of firm evidence of benefit. The practitioners of unorthodox methods may be very ethical and well meaning, but there are no safeguards to protect patients

The Risks of Alternative Treatments

- Many have not been scientifically tested, benefits are uncertain and side effects may be dangerous or may interfere with conventional treatments.
- Costs may be prohibitive and not covered by insurance.
- While some practitioners are honest and principled, others are not.
- If a rigorous diet or regimen shows no results, the person may feel a sense of personal failure with accompanying guilt that's damaging to self-esteem and can undermine health.
- A person with terminal cancer may spend a lot of time chasing dubious "cures," instead of coming to terms with the disease and making the best of the time left.
- Most crucial – reliance on alternative therapy may lead people to delay or ignore conventional treatment that has proven benefits.

from unprincipled "healers." Those who seek alternative therapies should ask about the methods used, and try to find practitioners with a reputation for honesty and reliability. Another problem is that if the cancer does not respond to a change, say, in behavior or diet, the person may feel like a failure. Many people already (mistakenly) feel responsible and guilty for getting cancer in the first place – due to some personal misdeed, neglect or stress in their lives. Although accepting responsibility in making treatment choices is essential, blaming oneself for a disease that's not one's fault can be soul-destroying and can undermine therapy.

Finally, some cancers are very treatable and can be cured with standard therapy. Although every woman has the right to choose from a full range of treatments, if she delays or refuses medical anti-cancer treatment in favor of unproven methods, her chances of being cured may be diminished or lost.

TWENTY

Prevention

Given the heavy toll of breast cancer and the dismal statistics – with death rates that have declined only slightly since the 1930s – prevention is a must. Scientists look to the possible causes of breast cancer to try to find ways to prevent it. But since the biology and causes of breast cancer are still incompletely understood, direct prevention is difficult. The much-publicized discovery of the BRCA1 and BRCA2 cancer-susceptibility genes, while a great credit to the researchers involved and a promise of future treatment or cure, does little to help women who have or are at risk of breast cancer today.

The current prevention strategies, such as they are, attempt to increase resistance or decrease susceptibility to the disease mainly by avoiding known or possible risk factors – such as post-menopausal obesity, high-fat diets and lack of exercise. Recently, drug trials have been initiated, giving tamoxifen or other hormonal agents to healthy women at high risk of the disease to see if it will prevent breast cancer from occurring – for example, in women with several close family members who

Recapping the Chief Known Risk Factors

Unmodifiable risk factors:

- *being female* (women have 100 times more breast cancer than men);
- *country of birth* (rates in North America and northern Europe are particularly high);
- *increasing age;*
- *very dense breast tissue* (as shown on a mammogram);
- *atypical benign hyperplasia* (breast tissue overgrowth containing atypical cells);
- *already having had cancer* in one breast;
- *a family history of the disease* – having close relatives (a mother, sister or grandmother) who had breast cancer early, particularly in both breasts;
- *predisposing genes* (for example, BRCA1 or BRCA2);
- *early onset of menstruation;*
- *late menopause.*

Modifiable risk factors:

- *having no children, or having them late,* after age 30;
- *obesity* (after menopause);
- *diet high in fat* and low in fruit and vegetables (possibly);
- *moderate alcohol consumption* (more than one to two drinks a day);
- *lack of vigorous physical activity,* especially at a young age (before or at puberty and into adolescence).

have or had the disease.

Re-examining the known causes and risk factors for breast cancer (described in Chapter ll) gives pointers to ways in which women might try to reduce the chance of getting it.

Trying to Change Alterable Risk Factors

While many of the risk factors for breast cancer are unalterable, women *can* modify alterable lifestyle factors to try to reduce the chances of getting breast cancer. Possible ways to decrease risks of breast cancer include eating a low-fat diet, limiting alcohol intake, getting enough vigorous exercise from an early age on, and avoiding post-menopausal obesity – strategies that may also decrease cardiovascular disease, the major killer of women.

Exploring the Diet-Cancer Connection
The risk of cancer in general can be diminished by avoiding known carcinogens (cancer-causing agents) such as tobacco products, ultraviolet rays and certain environmental toxins, and – according to the latest evidence – by limiting alcohol and dietary fat intake, and by eating plenty of fruit and vegetables.

Results from many recent studies link low intakes of fresh fruit and vegetables to high cancer rates. Some researchers claim that not eating enough fruits and vegetables *doubles* the risk of many forms of cancer, including breast cancer. Certain plant constituents in fruit and vegetables are thought to protect against cancer. (Studies also suggest that olive, canola and flaxseed oils may protect against breast and other cancers.) Since less than 10 percent of North Americans eat the recommended ten or more daily servings of fruit and vegetables, there's ample room for improvement.

Although epidemiological studies (which examine the distribution and risks of disease) cannot prove a *causal* relationship between diet and cancer, much can be learned by comparing cancer rates and lifestyles in various countries. For example, *breast cancer* is far more common in Canada than in Japan; *esophageal cancer* is far more frequent in Africa than in many parts of India; *stomach cancer* is 12 times more common in Japan than in Ibadan; *urinary bladder cancer* is 10 times more frequent in the U.S. than in India; *rectal cancer* is about 50 times more prevalent in Canada than in many parts of Africa. The comparisons suggest that certain factors in the diets of more developed nations lead to increased cancer rates. In general, populations that consume largely vegetarian diets have lower cancer rates than those who eat more meat and animal fat.

Significantly, when people migrate to a new country and adopt its lifestyle they soon acquire the same cancer rates as those born in the adopted country. For example, if Japanese people (who have low rates of breast and colon cancer but high rates of stomach cancer) move to the U.S., they acquire typical American cancer rates – high colon and breast cancer rates, low risks of stomach cancer.

Such findings reveal a picture of the diet-cancer link in which some dietary constituents promote certain cancers – such as fat (mainly from meat), excess energy (calories) and heavy alcohol consumption – while others, especially components in fruit and vegetables, may protect against cancer. Other elements that may protect against certain cancers include starch, fatty acids in fish (the N-3 or omega-3 fatty acids) and soya products (thought to protect against breast cancer in particular). Early research suggests that phytoestrogens in soya beans and flax seeds may block estrogen receptors in breast cells and inhibit the hormonal influences that promote tumor growth. Together, the plant components that seem to fight cancer have been dubbed "chemopreventive agents."

The Anti-Cancer Effects of Fruit and Veggies

The fruits and vegetables that appear most protective against cancer are raw, dark green leafy vegetables (such as spinach, kale and some lettuce), *cruciferous* or cabbage-family types (such as Brussels sprouts, cabbage, cauliflower and broccoli) and orange forms such as carrots, squash, citrus and other fruits. But it's best to eat more of all fruits and vegetables, to reduce the risk of cancer in general.

The Possible Anti-cancer Role of Antioxidants

The anti-cancer or "chemopreventive" effects of fruits and

vegetables are attributed by some to antioxidants, especially the carotenoids or vitamin-A precursors. The carotenoids are red, orange and yellow pigments found in a multitude of fruit and vegetables including sweet potatoes, apricots, cantaloupe, tomatoes, corn, carrots and peppers – and in dark green leafy vegetables. Some carotenoids are converted into active vitamin A (retinal) inside the body, others are not.

What about Vitamin Supplements?
Since antioxidants found in fruits and vegetables seem to reduce cancer risks, it's reasonable to wonder whether one should take supplements. While opinions vary, most nutritional scientists do *not* encourage the use of vitamin or other supplements for cancer prevention. People can easily obtain all essential nutrients from a healthy balanced diet. "Besides the risk of toxicity if people take megadoses, there is the added danger," notes one nutritionist, "that people who take vitamin supplements may falsely believe they are eating well, yet fail to achieve the health benefits of a well-balanced diet."

In other words, people who take supplements may be careless about eating the recommended quota of fruits and vegetables. Since we don't yet understand the nutritional role of all the substances in plants, they may miss out on other valuable components – perhaps get even less effective health protection. There may be plant constituents that, unknown to us, contribute to cancer prevention. The evidence for the anti-cancer benefits of antioxidant supplements is far less convincing than that for the known benefits of whole fresh fruit and vegetables.

There is also concern about the safety of antioxidant supplements. Although vitamins C, E and beta-carotene have low toxicity, even when consumed in doses far beyond recommended daily amounts, a few studies suggest that consuming large doses may not always be safe. For example, in animal experiments, beta-carotene supplements worsened the liver damage caused by alcohol consumption. There are also indications that large doses of beta-carotene may interfere with vitamin-E absorption by the body.

Reduce Obesity If Post-Menopausal

There is considerable evidence that obese older women have a doubled risk of breast cancer. This extra risk may possibly be due to the fact that fatty body tissues produce estrogens. Paradoxically, women often gain weight after a diagnosis of breast cancer, partly through overeating as a "comfort" strategy, and perhaps also because of some drug treatments, but weight gain in turn increases recurrence risks. "Sometimes," notes one oncologist, "the obesity is a sign of poor coping, and physicians and counselors can try to help women maintain or lose weight so they don't increase their recurrence risks."

Try Reducing Exposure to Estrogens

Female hormones play a key role in the origins of breast cancer, and may enhance tumor growth by increasing the speed of cell division. The modern Western tendency to an earlier menarche – onset of menstruation – and delayed childbearing may considerably increase women's susceptibility to breast cancer because of the added years of exposure to estrogen. The longer the gap between menarche and first childbirth, the greater the risk. In addition, since estrogen is used in birth-control pills and for post-menopausal hormone therapy, women in known high-risk categories should discuss the potential risks with their caregivers, especially in regard to the wisdom of taking menopausal hormone supplements. (See also Chapter 11.) While women cannot alter the age of menarche, they can perhaps *try* to have their children earlier rather than later in life; they can also breastfeed, which may help reduce the risks.

Genetic Tests for Those with a Family Predisposition

A test may soon become available for those in cancer-prone families to see if they are carrying cancer-susceptibility genes. As already mentioned, those considered to be at genetically high risk for breast cancer are women with two or more close family members who have or had breast cancer, particularly before menopause, especially if it affected both breasts. People from such families can seek specialized genetic counseling which may help reduce the understandable anxiety.

What about Drugs for Chemoprevention?

There are various clinical trials starting up for people known to be at high risk, to investigate a "chemopreventive" approach using various hormonal agents. One agent, a *gonadotropin-releasing hormone agonist* that blocks estrogen release, containing a low-dose estrogen and intermittent progestin, is being tried in a Los Angeles clinical trial. The second is the anti-estrogen drug tamoxifen, already described.

Tamoxifen is one of the few drugs available that can, in certain circumstances, reduce the occurrence of second primary breast cancers in women who have already had cancer in one breast. In the Breast Cancer Prevention Trial (BCPT) now under way in 270 centers in the U.S. and Canada, tamoxifen is being tested for its chemopreventive properties in healthy women known to be at high risk, to see if it can prevent the disease. The trial was temporarily halted when critics alleged that the women had not been told or adequately warned of potential side effects: hot flashes, eye problems, depression and, more seriously, increased risks of endometrial cancer. (Risks of endometrial cancer go up with the dose and years of tamoxifen use.) Updated consent forms have since been prepared and the trial continues.

Possible Ways to Reduce Breast Cancer Risks
In adults:
- reduce overall fat intake to 25 percent or less of total calories;
- substitute olive or canola oil for other fats (including corn oil);
- eat at least five to ten daily servings of widely varied fruit and vegetables;
- limit alcohol consumption;
- have regular, vigorous physical activity from early years and continue at least moderate exercise into the middle and later years;
- consider bearing children early if possible.

In daughters and granddaughters:
- make sure they eat a low-fat diet rich in fruit and vegetables and get plenty of vigorous exercise from an early age, during childhood and into adolescence (which may delay the onset of menstruation, hence reducing estrogen-exposure).

In Conclusion
Breast cancer is a ravaging disease that kills many women, sometimes within a few years of diagnosis, sometimes women with young children. It's also a disease that creates a deep emotional and psychosocial burden. It not only attacks breast tissue but also strikes at the very core of a woman's sense of self, her sexual image, gender role and nurturing ability. We desperately need better, gentler, less toxic treatments, and above all some means of prevention. But there is hope, and there are many long-term survivors. On my street, I know three women who had breast cancer 20 to 30 years ago. Each spring, as the snow melts, I see them emerge to plant their gardens, walk their dogs, play tennis, ride their bicycles and carry on with life.

Summing Up: Ways to Reduce Your Chances of Dying from Breast Cancer

- *Maintain desirable body weight.*
- *Avoid obesity,* especially after menopause.
- *Exercise regularly* and vigorously (and encourage daughters to do likewise), starting before adolescence, and continuing activity in middle age.
- *Reduce dietary fat* to 25 percent or less of total calories.
- *Select monounsaturated fats* (such as olive, flaxseed and canola oils) rather than saturated or polyunsaturated types.
- *Eat plenty (at least 5 to 10 daily servings) of fresh fruit and vegetables* – especially dark green leafy kinds, cabbage-family vegetables such as cauliflower, cabbage and broccoli, and bright orange forms such as cantaloupe, squash, carrots and citrus fruits.
- *Limit alcohol consumption.*
- *If planning to have children,* consider having them early in life, if possible, and consider breastfeeding for several months – which may reduce risks if done for a cumulative period of several years.
- *Have regular breast examinations* by a qualified health professional.
- *Get regular mammograms* after age 50 – and perhaps earlier if in a high-risk group.
- *Practice breast self-examination.*
- *If you have a strong family history* of breast cancer, get extra-frequent checkups and seek expert advice about prevention. Get genetic counseling.
- *Don't panic* if you think you see a sign of cancer. Remember that most breast problems are not cancerous. Even if cancer is present, prompt treatment may allow a complete cure. However bad the problem, it's far worse to have it unidentified – and growing bigger – without knowing or doing anything about it.

Glossary

Adjuvant therapy: Additional treatment given after surgery to prevent recurrence or further spread or growth of cancer cells, using radiation, cancer-killing drugs (chemotherapy) and/or hormone therapy.

Androgens: Male hormones used to slow or stop metastatic (secondary) tumor growth.

Areola: Area of pigmented skin around the nipple.

Atypical cells: Cells that appear abnormal but not cancerous under the microscope, sometimes a marker of possible future cancer development.

Autologous: From the patient's own body.

Axilla: The armpit area. "Axillary dissection" refers to removal of lymph nodes in the armpit area for diagnostic purposes.

Benign tumor: A growth or lump that is noncancerous.

Biopsy: Removal of a small sample of suspicious tissue, by needle or surgery, for microscopic examination.

Breast-conserving surgery: *See* Lumpectomy.

Breast implant: A round or teardrop-shaped sac (often saline-filled) implanted, sometimes under the skin, sometimes under the chest-wall muscle, to improve breast shape or size.

Breast reconstruction: Surgical procedures that create or reconstruct a breast mound and/or nipple after mastectomy, using the patient's own body tissues or a breast implant.

Breast self-examination (BSE): Monthly examination of breasts by the woman herself to find changes.

Calcifications: Tiny deposits of calcium in the breast tissue, seen on a mammogram, that may signify cancer.

Cancer: A term covering many different malignant diseases, characterized by DNA changes that disrupt the cells' normal regulatory processes with uncontrolled cell division that may invade and destroy surrounding tissues.

Carcinoma: Another word for cancer.

Carcinoma in situ: Cancer that remains localized and non-invasive – does not spread beyond the original site.

Chemotherapy: "Systemic" treatment with cell-killing drugs to destroy cancer cells throughout the body.

Clinical trials: Carefully designed scientific studies on people to test the efficacy of a drug, procedure or other treatment.

Cyst: A usually noncancerous fluid-filled sac.

Cytological: Cellular.

Cytotoxic: Cell-killing.

Diagnosis: Identification of a disease from its signs and symptoms.

Dissection: Surgical procedure that cuts open and separates tissues in any part of the body.

Ductal ectasia: Inflamed ducts.

Ducts: Tubes in the breast that carry milk from the lobes to the nipple.

Edema: Swelling of body tissues due to accumulation of fluid, a frequent problem after the axillary surgery that usually accompanies breast cancer operations.

Endocrine: Related to hormones; here referring to hormonal treatments for breast cancer.

Epidemiological: A branch of science that examines differences in disease rates in different countries or among different groups of people, to look for causes and trends.

Estrogen: A female hormone produced mainly by the ovaries (and in fat tissue) that triggers development of female breasts and other secondary female characteristics. Estrogen plays a key role in the menstrual cycle and stimulates the growth of some breast cancers.

Estrogen receptor (ER): A protein in the breast cell that binds to estrogen and helps it stimulate tissue and tumor growth. A cancer cell that is ER-positive has estrogen receptors and usually responds to anti-estrogen hormone therapy.

Fibroadenoma: A noncancerous breast lump.

Fine-needle aspiration (FNA): A biopsy technique in which a thin needle is inserted into a lump to withdraw fluid and/or a few cells for microscopic examination.

Fine-wire localization: A technique in which a fine wire is placed in the breast under mammographic control to guide the surgeon to the abnormal area to be removed.

Gene: A segment of the genetic material (DNA) inside the chromosomes in a cell nucleus, which controls protein production and hereditary traits.

Histological: Related to body tissues.

Hormone replacement therapy (HRT): Use of estrogen-progestin mixtures, after natural or surgically induced menopause, to reduce menopausal discomforts and post-menopausal health risks to bones and heart.

Hormone therapy: Treatment of breast cancer with agents that block the cancer-stimulating effects of estrogen or other hormones.

Hormones: Special chemical messengers produced by endocrine (hormone) glands that travel through the bloodstream to affect and stimulate certain "target" organs in the body. (For example, estrogen secreted by the ovaries causes menstrual-cycle changes.)

Hyperplasia: Noncancerous cell overgrowth.

Incidence: The number of new cases of a specific disease diagnosed per year in a given population.

In-situ cancer: *See* Carcinoma in situ.

Invasive cancer: Cancer that has spread from its original site to invade adjacent tissues.

Large-core needle biopsy: Withdrawal of tissue samples from the breast using a special large-core needle.

Lobules: The milk-producing or glandular parts of the breast.

Lumpectomy: Surgical procedure to remove a cancerous breast tumor with a margin of surrounding normal breast tissue (also called "partial mastectomy" or "breast-conserving surgery").

Lymph nodes: Small, bean-shaped structures that act as filters to inactivate microorganisms and defend against infection. Underarm lymph nodes are often removed in breast cancer operations, to be tested for cancer.

Lymphatic system: The network of vessels that drains lymph fluid from tissues of the body.

Lymphedema: Swelling of the arm and armpit area after breast surgery, which can be uncomfortable and may recur, requiring drainage and other strategies. (*See also* Edema.)

Malignant: Cancerous.

Mammogram: A low-dose breast X-ray used to evaluate and diagnose abnormalities in the breast, or to find abnormalities in healthy women who as yet show no symptoms.

Markers: Molecular or biochemical features of a tumor identified by the pathologist and used to help type and stage the cancer and predict its behavior.

Mastectomy: Surgical removal of the breast.

Medical oncologist: Physician who specializes in drug therapy (chemotherapy) for cancer.

Menarche: Onset of menstruation (periods).

Menopause: Time of life around age 50 to 52 when a woman's eggs are used up or stop ripening and menstrual periods cease, with a drop in the secretion of estrogen.

Metastasis: The spread of cancer cells from the original (primary) tumor through the bloodstream or lymphatic system to other body sites.

Microcalcifications: Very tiny specks of calcium, visible on a mammogram, that may signify the presence of cancer.

Modified radical mastectomy: A breast cancer operation that removes breast and underarm nodes but no muscle. *See* Radical mastectomy.

Morbidity: The sickness, handicap, disability or unwellness caused by a disease.

Mortality: Deaths attributable to a given illness or condition; the mortality rate is the number of deaths due to that condition in a given number of people in a given time.

Mutation: A change in a gene (segment of DNA) that can lead to abnormal cell function or disease.

Necrosis: The death of cells in some part of the body's tissue, or within a malignant tumor.

Oncogenes: Genes involved in suppressing or triggering cancer.

Oncologist: A physician or surgeon who specializes in treating cancer.

Palpation: Examination of the body with the hands, to feel what's under the skin. A "palpable" lesion is a clearly felt lump, thickening or change.

Partial mastectomy: *See* Lumpectomy.

Pathologist: A physician who specializes in identifying diseases by examining the structure of cells and tissues.

Pectoral muscles: Muscles of the chest.

Plastic surgeon: A surgeon who specializes in reconstructive or cosmetic surgery – including breast reconstruction.

Prevalence: The number of cases of a disease found in a given population at a given point in time.

Primary cancer: A tumor in the site where it originated, as opposed to a "secondary tumor" caused by cells that have escaped from the primary tumor to form tumors elsewhere.

Progesterone: A female hormone produced by the ovaries in the second half of the menstrual cycle, and by the placenta in pregnancy, which can stimulate growth of some breast cancers.

Prognosis: The predicted course or outcome of a disease.

Prognostic factors: Characteristics that help foretell a cancer's behavior – whether it is aggressive (fast-dividing), has certain cell receptors and so on – used to predict the probability of recurrence and survival.

Prophylactic: Preventive treatment that can involve many strategies, e.g., diet changes, drugs, surgery, radiation.

Prosthesis: An artificial breast form or device worn in or under clothing to create a "normal-looking" breast after mastectomy.

Radiation oncologist: A physician who specializes in treating cancer with radiation.

Radical mastectomy: Removal of the breast along with some chest muscles and underarm nodes.

Radiologist: A physician trained in X-ray and other imaging techniques (such as ultrasound or magnetic resonance imaging).

Radiotherapy (or radiation therapy): The use of ionizing radiation (e.g., X-rays and electrons) to shrink tumors and kill outlying cancer cells.

Reconstruction (mammoplasty): Re-creation of a breast that's been removed.

Recurrence: The return of cancer growth, at the original site (local recurrence) or elsewhere (systemic or distant recurrence), after a "disease-free" spell when there was no evidence of the cancer.

Risk factor: A factor that increases the chances of getting cancer, either genetic (inherited), environmental (such as air pollution, DDT) or lifestyle (such as diet).

Screening: Testing for unsuspected early disease in healthy people who have no symptoms of the disease.

Secondary cancer: A cancer that has spread from the original (primary) site to another site (also called metastatic cancer). Secondary tumors may retain the characteristics of the primary cancer, even though they appear in other parts of the body.

Segmental mastectomy: *See* Lumpectomy.

Staging: Establishing the extent, invasiveness and likely spread of a cancer.

Subcutaneous: Beneath the skin.

Sutures: Stitches (sometimes self-dissolving or disposable) used to close surgical wounds.

Systemic: Affecting the entire body, not just one specific part.

Tamoxifen: An anti-estrogen that blocks the growth-stimulating effects of estrogen on cancer cells – frequently used in treating breast cancer.

Tumor: Abnormal tissue growth that can be malignant (cancerous) or benign (noncancerous).

Ultrasonography (ultrasound): A non-invasive imaging technique using high-frequency sound waves converted to images on a screen, used to view internal parts of the body.

White blood cells: Infection-fighting cells that destroy "foreign" material and abnormal (cancer) cells.

Wide-excision surgery: Surgery to remove a cancerous breast tumor and a wide rim of surrounding tissue.

Further Resources

Support and service organizations

The following organizations offer information, assistance and emotional support to people living with cancer, and their families, on a national basis, through local chapters.

Canada (National)

Alliance of Breast Cancer
  Survivors
P.O. Box 2035
20 Eglinton Avenue West
Toronto, ON M4R 1K8
(416) 487-9899
Fax (416) 487-0584

Breast Cancer Action
P.O. Box 4332
Station E
Ottawa, ON K1S 5B3
(613) 736-5921

Breast Cancer Information
  Exchange Project
Preventive Health Services
  Division
Health Canada

Jeanne Mance Bldg.,
  Room 641
Tunney's Pasture
Ottawa, ON K1A 1B4
(613) 954-8668
Fax (613) 941-2633

Canadian Breast Cancer
  Foundation
620 University Avenue,
  7th Floor
Toronto, ON M5S 2C1
(416) 596-6773
1-800-387-9816

Canadian Breast Cancer Network
P.O. Box 45115
2482 Yonge Street
Toronto, ON M4P 2H0
(416) 244-1443
Fax (416) 244-2363

Canadian Cancer Society
10 Alcorn Avenue,
   Suite 200
Toronto, ON M4V 3B1
(416) 961-7223

Cancer Information Service
1-800-263-6750

Consumer Health
   Information Service
1-800-667-1999

Mission Air Transportation
   Network
For address see Canadian Cancer
   Society, above.
(Nation-wide program to give
   patients with cancer the use of
   available seats on corporate
   aircraft.)

Ontario Cancer Treatment and
   Research Foundation
620 University Avenue
Toronto, ON M5G 2L7
(416) 971-9800
Fax (416) 971-6888

"Wellspring" (Support Group)
The Coach House
81 Wellesley Street East
Toronto, ON M4Y 1H6
(416) 961-1928
Fax (416) 961-3721

Willow
Breast Cancer Support and
   Resource Center
519 Jarvis Str., 2nd Floor
Toronto, ON M4Y 1H7
(416) 926-4537
Fax (416) 926-6521

Provincial

Alberta
Alberta Cancer Board
9707–110 Street, 6th Floor
Edmonton, AB T5K 2L9
(403) 782-3491

Breast Cancer Info Link
   (Prairies/NWT)
1331–29 Street NW
Calgary, AB T2N 4N2
(403) 670-2113
Fax (403) 283-1651

Canadian Cancer Society
Alberta/NWT
2424 4th Street SW, 2nd Floor
Calgary, AB T2S 2T4
(403) 228-4487

Cross Cancer Institute
11560 University Avenue
Edmonton, AB T6G 1Z2
(403) 432-8763

Tom Baker Cancer Centre
1331 29th Street NW
Calgary, AB T2N 4N2
(403) 270-1700

British Columbia
BC/Yukon Breast Cancer
    Info Project
For address see Canadian Cancer
    Society, British
    Columbia/Yukon, below.

Canadian Cancer Society
British Columbia/Yukon
565 West 10th Avenue
Vancouver, BC V5Z 4J4
(604) 872-4400

Cancer Control Agency of
    British Columbia
600 West 10th Avenue
Vancouver, BC V5Z 4E6
(604) 877-6000

Victoria Cancer Clinic
1900 Fort Street
Victoria, BC V8R 1J8

Manitoba
Canadian Cancer Society
193 Sherbrook Street
Winnipeg, MB R3C 2B7
(204) 774-7483

Manitoba Cancer Treatment and
    Research Foundation
100 Olivia Street
Winnipeg, MB R3E 0V9
(204) 787-2271

New Brunswick
Canadian Cancer Society
P.O. Box 2089
63 Union Street
Saint John, NB E2L 3T5
(506) 634-6272

Newfoundland & Labrador
Canadian Cancer Society
P.O. Box 8921
Chimo Building, 1st Floor
St. John's, NF A1B 3R9
(709) 753-6520

Newfoundland Cancer Clinic
Health Sciences Centre
Prince Philip Drive
St. John's, NF A1B 3V6
(709) 737-6439

Newfoundland Cancer Treatment
    and Research Foundation
25 Kenmount Road
St. John's, NF A1B 1W1

Nova Scotia
Canadian Cancer Society
5826 South Street, Suite 1
Halifax, NS B3H 1S6
(902) 423-6183

Cancer Treatment and Research
    Foundation of Nova Scotia
5820 University Avenue
Halifax, NS B3H 1V7
(902) 428-4209

Ontario
Breast Cancer Information and
    Education Services
51 Hillcrest Avenue
St. Catharines, ON
    L2R 4Y3
(905) 687-3333

Burlington Breast Cancer
    Support Service
777 Guelph Line
Burlington, ON L7R 3N2
(416) 634-2333

Canadian Cancer Society
1639 Yonge Street
Toronto, ON M4T 2W6
(416) 488-5400

Cancer Counselling Centre
Toronto, ON
(416) 778-4657

Connecting Rainbows
c/o 109 Booth Drive
Stouffville, ON L4A 4S1
(905) 642-2329

Helping You Helps Me
244 Hugel Avenue
Midland, ON L4R 1T2
(705) 527-6278

Mind over Cancer
53 Gillespie Crescent
Ottawa, ON K1V 0W2
(613) 738-1017

Ontario Cancer Institute
Princess Margaret Hospital
500 Sherbourne Street
Toronto, ON M4X 1K9
(416) 924-0671

Thunder Bay Regional
    Cancer Centre
290 Munro Street
Thunder Bay, ON P7A 7T1
(807) 343-1610
Fax (807) 345-2030

Toronto-Bayview Sunnybrook
    Cancer Centre
2075 Bayview Avenue
Toronto, ON M4N 3M5
(416) 488-5801
Fax (416) 480-6002

Prince Edward Island
Atlantic Breast Cancer
    Information Project
1 Rochford St., Suite 1
Charlottetown, PEI C1A 3T1
(902) 892-9531
Fax (902) 628-8281

Canadian Cancer Society
P.O. Box 115
Charlottetown, PEI C1A 7K2
(902) 566-4007

Department of Health and
 Social Services
Oncology Division
P.O. Box 2000
Charlottetown, PEI C1A 7P1
(902) 522-6027

Quebec
Breast Cancer Action
5890 Monkland, Suite 203
Montreal, QC H4A 1G2
(514) 483-1846
Fax (514) 482-1445

Canadian Cancer Society
5151, boul. l'Assomption
Montreal, QC H1T 4A9
(514) 255-5151

Quebec Breast Cancer
 Information Project
3840 Rue Saint Urbain
Montreal, QC H2W 1T8
(514) 843-2930

Saskatchewan
Allan Blair Memorial Clinic
4101 Dewdney Avenue
Regina, SK S4T 7T1
(306) 766-2333

Canadian Cancer Society
201–2445 13th Avenue
Regina, SK S4P 0W1
(306) 757-4260

Saskatchewan Cancer Foundation
2631 28th Avenue
Regina, SK S4S 6X3
(306) 585-1831

U.S. (National)
American Association for
 Cancer Education
MD Anderson Cancer Center
151 Holcombe Boulevard
Houston, TX 77030
(713) 792-3020
Fax (713) 792-0807

American Cancer Society (ACS)
1599 Clifton Road NE
Atlanta, GA 30329
(800) ACS-2345
(404) 320-3333
Fax (404) 325-0230

Breast Cancer Advisory
 Center (BCAC)
P.O. Box 224
Kensington, MD 20895
Fax (301) 949-1132

Cancer Care
1180 Avenue of the Americas
New York, NY 10036
(212) 221-3300

Cancer Control Society (CCS)
2043 N. Berendo Street
Los Angeles, CA 90027
(213) 663-7801

Cancer Information Service
Office of Cancer Information
NCI/NIH, Building 31, 10A07
9000 Rockville Pike
Bethesda, MD 20892
(800) 4-CANCER
Fax (301) 402-0555

Candelighters Childhood
   Cancer Foundation
7910 Woodmont Ave.,
   Suite 460
Bethesda, MD 20814-3015
(800) 366-2223
Fax (301) 718-2686

National Alliance of Breast
   Cancer Organizations
   (NABCO)
9 E. 37th St., 10th Floor
New York, NY 10016
(212) 719-0154
Fax (212) 689-1213

National Coalition for Cancer
   Survivorship (NCCS)
1010 Wayne Ave., 5th Floor
Silver Spring, MD 20910
(301) 650-8868
Fax (301) 565-9670

Patient Advocates for
   Advanced Cancer Treatment
1143 Parmelee NW
Grand Rapids, MI 49504-3844
(616) 453-1477
Fax (616) 453-1846

Reach to Recovery
c/o American Cancer Society,
   see above

Susan G. Komen Breast
   Cancer Foundation
5005 LBJ, Suite 370
Dallas, TX 75244
(800) TM-AWARE
Fax (214) 450-1710

Y-ME National Breast
   Cancer Organization
212 W. Van Buren
Chicago, IL 60607
(800) 221-2141
Fax (312) 986-0020

Networking, advocacy and activism centres across North America

Alliance of Breast Cancer Survivors
20 Eglinton Avenue West,
   Suite 1106
Toronto, ON M4R 1K8
(416) 487-9899
Fax (416) 487-0584

Bayview Support Network
c/o Toronto Bayview Cancer
   Centre
2075 Bayview Avenue
Toronto, ON M4N 3M5
(416) 480-6898

NABCO, National Alliance of
   Breast Cancer Organizations
1180 Avenue of the Americas,
   2nd Floor
New York, NY
U.S.A. 10036
(212) 719-0154

National Coalition for Cancer
   Survivorship
1010 Wayne Avenue, 5th Floor
Silver Spring, MD
U.S.A. 20910
(301) 650-8868

Y-ME National Association for
   Breast Cancer Information
   and Support
18220 Harwood Avenue
Homewood, IL
U.S.A. 60430
(709) 799-8228

Books

Batt, Sharon. 1994. *Patient No More*. Gynergy Books.

Baum, M., C. Saunders, & S. Meredith. 1993. *Breast Cancer*. Oxford University Press.

Boston Women's Health Collective. 1992. *The New Our Bodies, Ourselves: A Book by and for Women*. Simon and Schuster.

Brinker, Nancy. 1990. *The Race Is Run One Step at a Time – Everywoman's Guide to Taking Charge of Breast Cancer*. Fireside–Simon and Schuster.

Community Cancer Resource Guide. 1995. From Toronto-Bayview Sunnybrook Cancer Centre, 2075 Bayview Avenue, Toronto, ON M4W 3M5. For information call (416) 480-4662 or fax (416) 480-6876.

Dackman, Linda. 1990.
Up Front – Sex and Post-Mastectomy Woman. Viking.

Gross, Amy, & Ito Dee. 1991. *Women Talking about Breast Surgery.* HarperPerennial.

Kushner, Rose. 1985.
Alternatives, New Developments in the War on Breast Cancer. Warner.

Love, Dr. Susan M. 1990. *Dr. Susan Love's Breast Book.* Addison Wesley.

Olivotto, I., K. Gelmon, & V. Kuusk. *Breast Cancer.* Patient Guides.

A Guide to Unconventional Cancer Therapies. 1995. R&R Book Bar, 14800 Yonge Street, Unit 106, Aurora, ON L4S 1N3. Call (416) 480-5899 or (905) 727-3300 for information.

Siegel, Dr. B. S. 1989. *Peace, Love & Healing.* Harper & Row.

Williams, Penelope. 1993. *That Other Place: A Personal Account of Breast Cancer.* Dundurn.

Alternative Medicine: Expanding Medical Horizons, A Report to the National Institutes of Health. 1992. For information call (202) 512-1800, or fax (202) 512-2250.

Tapes

Voices in the Night. A Cancer Companion. From the Recovery Resource Centre, 1853 Grant Avenue, Winnipeg, MB R3W 2B1. For information, call 1-800-268-0009.

Breast Self-Examination. 1995. Ontario Cancer Institute. For information call (416) 924-0671.

Index

To the Reader

YOUR PERSONAL HEALTH SERIES is developed with the Canadian Medical Association and will encompass more than 20 subjects. The first six publications are *Migraine, Eyes, Arthritis, Sleep, Crohn's Disease and Ulcerative Colitis* and *The Complete Breast Book*.

If you wish to be kept informed about the series, please complete and send us this page (or a photocopy). We will be pleased to send you periodic publication notices on new and forthcoming titles.

Key Porter Books Limited
70 The Esplanade
Toronto, Ontario M5E 1R2 Canada
Telephone (416) 862-7777 • Fax (416) 862-2304

☐ Please keep me informed about YOUR PERSONAL HEALTH SERIES

☐ Please ship and bill____copy/ies of each new book upon publication

_____
NAME

_____
AFFILIATION (COMPANY/ASSOCIATION/INSTITUTION/MEDICAL AFFILIATION)

_____
ADDRESS

_____
CITY/TOWN   PROVINCE   POSTAL CODE

PAYMENT BY: ☐ VISA   ☐ MASTERCARD

_____
CREDIT CARD NO.

_____
EXPIRY DATE

_____
SIGNATURE

☐ Please invoice to above

Publication prices will vary and are subject to change without notice. GST and shipping and handling charges will be added to the invoice.